Clinical Pragmatics

To our families   Perheillemme
Beryl and Stan Haddleton
Irja, Heikki ja Markku Leinonen

And to the memory of Stan Basil Broadbent

Clinical Pragmatics
Unravelling the complexities of communicative failure

Benita Rae Smith

Department of Speech Pathology
Leicester Polytechnic

and

Eeva Leinonen

Department of Linguistics
Hatfield Polytechnic
Watford

CHAPMAN & HALL
London · New York · Tokyo · Melbourne · Madras

Published by Chapman & Hall, 2–6 Boundary Row, London SE1 8HN

Chapman & Hall, 2–6 Boundary Row, London SE1 8HN, UK

Chapman & Hall, 29 West 35th Street, New York NY10001, USA

Chapman & Hall Japan, Thomson Publishing Japan, Hirakawacho Nemoto Building, 7F, 1-7-11 Hirakawa-cho, Chiyoda-ku, Tokyo 102, Japan

Chapman & Hall Australia, Thomas Nelson Australia, 102 Dodds Street, South Melbourne, Victoria 3205, Australia

Chapman & Hall India, R. Seshadri, 32 Second Main Road, CIT East, Madras 600 035, India

First edition 1992

© 1992 Benita Rae Smith and Eeva Leinonen

Typeset in 10/12 pt Palatino by Excel Typesetters, Hong Kong
Printed in Great Britain by Page Bros, Norwich

ISBN 0 412 34740 7

A catalogue record for this book is available from the British Library

Library of Congress Cataloging-in-Publication data

Smith, Benita Rae, 1934–
    Clinical pragmatics : unravelling the complexities of
communicative failure / Benita Rae Smith and Eeva Leinonen.
        p.   cm.
    Includes bibliographical references and index.
    1. Speech disorders.   2. Speech therapy.   3. Communicative
disorders.   I. Leinonen, Eeva, 1958–   . II. Title
    [DNLM: 1. Communicative Disorders.   2. Language Disorders.
3. Speech Disorders.   WL 340 S643c]
    RC423.S57   1991 /992
    616.85′5—dc20
DNLM/DLC
for Library of Congress   91–20759
                                                              CIP

Contents

Acknowledgements

Our thanks are due to Jennifer Eastwood, Lucie Andersen and Di Gordon for commenting on earlier drafts of certain chapters. Vicky Crawford and the Central Services Department at Leicester Polytechnic gave valuable assistance in the preparation of typescripts. Past and present students, who have confirmed our opinion that this book needed to be written, have also helped to shape our views while writing it and have motivated us to continue. Finally, many thanks are due to Terri Cooper and Tim Hardwick for commissioning and nurturing our work and to our partners Colin and Peter for enhancing our personal lives despite the trials of prolonged authorship. Lastly, thank you Angela for helping us to keep clinical pragmatics in perspective.

Preface

In setting out to write this book we were aware of the
confused and confusing subject area of pragmatic failure
and of some existing attempts to bring it under control.
We realized that clarification was necessary if clinicians,
students or any professionals involved in the exploration
of communication problems were to benefit from the wealth
of information and theory now available. We realized, at
the same time, that our own thinking was likely to remain
confused in certain areas due to the enormity of the task
we had set ourselves. No apology is made for this state of
affairs since others will undoubtedly improve upon our
efforts, now that some ground clearing has begun.

We also soon came to realize that certain important areas
had to be neglected in favour of others, given the constraints of a single volume. Pragmatic issues in comprehension are mentioned throughout, but not discussed in
the detail they deserve. Other areas which are only fleet-
ingly mentioned and which are of prime importance for a
volume on clinical pragmatics are those of intonation and
paralinguistics.

What we have attempted to do is to identify some key
concepts, explain these for those not familiar with pragmatic and discourse issues and explore links with the clinical practice of speech pathology and related disciplines.

Chapter 1 provides a broad overview of the process of
communication. It briefly explores the role of language,
intention, pragmatic principles, the channel, cognition and
psychological and social variables in the formulation, expression and interpretation of communicative behaviours.
By attempting to map out an overall picture of the various

influences affecting the creation of meaning in communication, we hope to emphasize, from the outset, the complexity of the phenomenon under discussion, thus attempting to guard our subsequent efforts from oversimplification.

In Chapter 2 we focus on how knowledge of pragmatics and discourse analysis enables one to examine communicative phenomena in general and in the speech and language pathology context in particular. The study of pragmatics has been shaped by philosophical, semiotic and linguistic influences providing different bases for investigating meaning in context. The idea of 'clinical pragmatics' as an area of 'applied pragmatics' is also introduced in this chapter and explored further in Chapter 4.

Chapter 3 is rather long, but, we feel, useful for those not familiar with the fields of pragmatics and discourse analysis. We aim to overview as clearly and succinctly as possible various key areas of study which have direct relevance for exploring the complexities of communicative success and failure. Ten areas of study are focused upon, carefully illustrating both what these areas mean and how they might prove useful for exploring the nature of communicative disturbance and failure. A section on clinical interaction is also included in order to illustrate how discourse analytical methods can be used for examining and evaluating not only the communicative behaviours of clients but also all participants. It is emphasized that the creation of meaningful and enjoyable interactions is a joint enterprise of all the participants.

If a field of study called 'clinical pragmatics' existed, what kinds of issues might it address? Chapter 4 provides a modest framework for clinical pragmatic study. It discusses issues relevant for identification, description and explanation of communicative behaviours. The issue of (in)appropriateness is a central one when considering communicative breakdown: indeed this is the very core of failing communications. It is paramount to consider from whose point of view, in which situations and for which reasons is one's communicative performance judged unacceptable and inappropriate. Three separate examples are discussed to illustrate various issues in clinical pragmatics.

In Chapter 5 we review the literature concerning disturbed pragmatic functioning, particularly in childhood, and discuss a method of conceptualizing these problems which may refine clinicians' categorizations and reveal the treatment needs of individuals within a widely heterogeneous group which, it may be said, has previously suffered from some rather unsatisfactory labelling.

With the above aims in mind, Chapter 6 examines available assessment materials. We do not claim to know which approaches ought to be used in specific cases and have not therefore attempted to advise clinicians in their selection of materials. What we have provided is a wide-ranging set of descriptions of available assessment methods with some evaluative comments.

A detailed treatment chapter dealing with the pragmatics-based remediation of a variety of communicative disorders was prepared, but was omitted for two reasons. It was felt that recommendations without the backing of 'effectiveness research' might not be helpful and that many of the approaches which we have found successful depend for their effectiveness upon a specific type of empowering relationship between clinician and client. With this in mind, Chapter 7 describes some of the obstacles which can impede clients' full participation in the process of recovery and some of the attitudes on the part of clinicians which can facilitate this participation. It is stressed that clients may be able to initiate and enjoy interactions when clinicians pay attention to the content of the clients' messages as well as their form and when clinicians avoid compulsive initiation and instruction.

Many of the principles discussed in Chapter 7 are illustrated in action in the brief case studies in Chapter 8. Four child clients are presented with special reference to their successful pragmatic development and to the part which shows awareness of functional communication played in the treatment of their varying communicative problems.

Chapter 9 sums up the implications of pragmatic approaches for the clinical management of communicative failure and for delivery of remedial services.

During the period of preparation of Clinical Pragmatics, more and more work has appeared which suggests that what we have been writing about may be a function of the right hemisphere of the human brain. While we have not

addressed the role of the right hemisphere in the processing of connected discourse and in the creation of meaning,
significance and emotional tone, we wish to stress the
potential value of pragmatically informed investigations.
Ellis and Young (1988:258) have the following to say about,
what they refer to as, 'high level impairment': 'What we
badly need before we can do proper cognitive neuropsychology is to know which of these impairments . . . can be
dissociated from which of the others, and which apparently co-occur. When we have such data we can begin to
speculate about the precise nature of the "high level"
language processing components which reside in the right
hemisphere, and we can begin to relate the impairments
of the right hemisphere injured patients to information-
processing models.' It is to endeavours such as these, as
well as to day to day clinical practice, that some of the
thinking presented in this volume may be able to make
a contribution.

Chapter 1

Exploring communication

Using concepts and methods employed in the fields of discourse analysis and pragmatics, we aim to explore communicative ability and disability. Communication is a truly complex phenomenon. The identification and description of communicative behaviours, the exploration of their appropriacy or inappropriacy, ventures into 'the murky realms of pragmatics' (Faerch and Kasper, 1983). We aim to dispense with some of the murkiness associated with the study of pragmatics, by demonstrating its usefulness and centrality in the clinical management of communication disorders. Communication can be studied not only as a collection of components within the 'scientific' paradigms of linguistics, psychology, speech pathology and medicine, but also within a paradigm of pragmatics which encompasses methods and principles for studying the whole of the communicative event rather than its separate components. The approach adopted here, that of clinical pragmatics (Chapter 2), considers the skills and abilities, the motivations and influences, which shape the communicative event both from the speaker/senders' and the listener/receivers' perspectives. Owing to the complexity of the phenomenon under discussion and the nature of our professional experience, not all relevant aspects of the communicative event are given equal emphasis and consideration. Leaving some loose ends and unanswered questions can only advance and stimulate thinking in the field of study which is still at an early stage of development. The 'pragmatics revolution' is now sweeping the speech therapy and speech pathology literature and is filtering into the practice of speech therapy. It is time to explore the nature of this 'revolution', its methods and procedures, and its strengths and weaknesses, for the clinical management of communication problems.

LANGUAGE AND COMMUNICATION

Speech-language professionals have the skills for describing clients' linguistic behaviours and linguistic systems. The field of linguistics has offered the practising clinicians many useful methods and procedures (and undoubtedly, many less useful ones too) for the description of the clients' phonetic, phonological, syntactic and semantic abilities and disabilities. An invasion of acronyms – LARSP, PRISM, PROPH, PROP, PACS, to mention but few – has provided clinicians with principled means of describing the client's linguistic ability and disability. The principles are based on linguistic theory (Crystal, 1981). The connection between linguistic theory and the clients' ability to share meanings in communication is not necessarily a direct one, and remains to be critically examined and evaluated (Chapter 4). Yet, assessment of client's language abilities constitutes an important part of the clinical assessment battery. The clients' productive and receptive capabilities can be mapped out as a function of articulatory (phonetic) or auditory ability. The use of sounds for the signalling of meaning differences in language can be explored in relation to phonological systems and patternings. The ability to vary tone, pitch, rhythm and intonation to signal meanings can also be considered an aspect of one's phonological knowledge. Knowing the meanings of words and combining words into meaningful sentences and utterances involves semantic and syntactic ability.

Undoubtedly, the very core of verbal communication involves these abilities to produce and comprehend language. Yet, such language abilities are only part of communicative ability. A great variety of non-verbal signals not only combine with language expressions to create meanings but also replace language altogether. At times it is not possible to convey meanings by using words: a nod across a crowded room might signal that it's time to leave, a smile approval, a frown disapproval and so on. And there are also people with little or no access to language who have the need to function, and can function, as communicators. Over-emphasis on language as a medium of communication can be unrealistic in the clinical context.

Not only is it necessary to explore one's linguistic knowledge as reflected in the various areas of linguistic analysis, but it also needs to be considered how these various aspects of knowledge interact in language use. It is not random or haphazard that a particular linguistic expression, pronunciation pattern, gesture or sign is chosen to express a particular meaning. Which meanings are expressed and how, whether verbally and/or non-verbally, depends on many factors beyond linguistic ones. At one level, meaning expressions may be constrained by motor problems. Quite simply, there may not be the motor abilities available for the articulation of the necessary sounds or sound sequences or for the expression of meanings via gestures and other bodily movements. Similarly, culture, sub-culture and educational experiences may promote or restrict certain communicative behaviours. The context in which the communicative event occurs also shapes the event: communicative behaviours may vary due to the nature of the communicative situation (e.g. formal vs. informal), the relationships of the participants, the purpose of the interaction and other such 'pragmatic' considerations. The age, sex and status of our communicative partner may promote the production of respectful, simplified, domineering and flirtatious language. Our perception of our interlocuter's ability to hear, see and process verbal and non-verbal expressions of meaning constrains our choices too, as does the assessment of the other person's knowledge of the world and language (our presuppositions). There are numerous influences which create, constrain and restrict the expression of meaning and which require careful consideration in the clinical context in order to avoid misassessment and misdiagnosis.

Language expressions do not exist in a vacuum: they are part of a whole communicative event. At times, it serves a purpose to separate language from communication, and study language ability/disability in such decontextualized terms; but to be able to assess what it is that makes a client unable to communicate meanings successfully, language needs to be considered as part of wider communication (Chapters 4, 5 and 6). Adopting a functional approach to language disability does not entail abandoning detailed analysis of language systems. What one is often faced with, however, is what to do with such analysis: what are the motivations for introducing one structure before another into the client's linguistic repertoire? A functional approach considers those aspects of one's linguistic system which appear most detrimental to the signalling of meanings in communication as priorities for treatment (Chapter 4).

There is a shift from looking at language ability/disability at separate linguistic levels to considering the client's ability to communicate and interact with others. This shift also encompasses interest in the interaction of linguistic levels and the effect of this interaction on communicative success (Crystal, 1987, Leinonen-Davies, 1988a; Chapter 4). It is not enough in communicative encounters to be able to produce intelligible utterances, it is also necessary to link these utterances to form longer stretches of language which in turn need to be coherent and relevant to the topic and the communicative context (Chapter 3). When interacting with others, we also need to be able to co-ordinate our contributions with our communicative partners in order to avoid speaking at the same time or to avoid uncomfortable silences. The study of communication requires a multidisciplinary approach. In the clinical context all aspects of communication are relevant, even if not equally important to every client. It is necessary to explore the various components of communicative behaviour and ability, in order to aid diagnosis, assessment and remediation.

The fields of 'discourse analysis' and 'pragmatics' address at communication entails beyond linguistic description nguage. The terms 'discourse' and 'pragmatics' are to describe a wide variety of phenomena. In broad te 'discourse' refers to interrelatedness and structuring ideas in conversation and texts (Coulthard, 1985) and matics' emphasizes intention, implicature, presuppo n and interpretation in the use of language (Levins 1983; Chapter 2). They are terms which are currently fashionable and easily roll off the tongue to describe many different phenomena which we find otherwise difficult to label. As long as such use serves a communicative purpose by describing the phenomena meaningfully and uniquely, we are not led too severely astray. However, in the context of speech pathology and therapy, the ability to identify and describe the communicative phenomena unambiguously and exhaustively and the ability to discuss it meaningfully are vital. A comprehensive description of communicative events is a tall order, so varied and numerous are the influences shaping the event, yet a great deal of order and pattern can be found and described. The fields of discourse analysis and pragmatics provide some of the means for exploring the patterns and behaviours in human communication. We shall explore the terms 'discourse analysis' and 'pragmatics' in more detail in Chapter 2 and concentrate here on what communication entails: on the substance of study for discourse analysis and pragmatics.

INTENTION IN COMMUNICATION

Communication is based on the notion of intentionality (e.g. de Beaugrande and Dressler, 1981). All meaning expressions (1) stem from the basic intention to participate and co-operate in a communicative interaction and (2) reflect the intention to convey certain meanings and not others. Let us consider these in more detail.

The basic motivations for participating in a communicative encounter derive from the need to survive (be fed, clothed, housed etc.) and the need for human contact. All people have these needs and consequently require some means of communicating with others. It is part of one's communicative ability to recognize one's needs and to plan and execute communicative behaviours in order to satisfy these needs. Such goals can range from buying some food, to telling someone how important they are to one, to talking about the weather with one's neighbour. While communication can be driven in a purposeful manner, much of it can be based on one being expected to communicate rather than really having the need to or wanting to do so. At times, one is expected to engage in communication and this expectation may not coincide with one's needs. This is likely to have consequences for the nature, effectiveness and enjoyment of the communicative event. In such expected communication, meanings with little significance for either partner are often expressed. In fact, the meaning which is often most clearly expressed, usually non-verbally and most likely unintentionally, is that of not wanting to communicate. Being expected to communicate is part of everyday life, and very early in life one learns the dynamics of these kinds of communicative encounters.

In the clinical context, the clinician and the client may feel that they are expected to communicate without a genuine desire to do so. The very nature of a clinical encounter, with a predetermined time, place and goals, is likely to shape the nature of the communicative event (Letts, 1985; Chapter 3). The principal aim of 'tightly structured' speech therapy (Chapter 7) is to improve the client's voice, articulation and language skills in the clinical setting. The tasks and exercises tend not to be based on communicative needs but on the 'needs' of the client's linguistic systems. The emphasis tends to be on how to bring the client's linguistic capabilities in line with those of 'normally functioning' individuals. Within this context, communicating in order to make something, for which there is a need, happen is not a top priority. Such communicative behaviours which are based on fairly fixed role models and fixed expectations can bear little resemblance to other communicative situations, and can thus hinder generalization of skill beyond the clinical context. Communication within a rigid model and without real purpose is no fun either; enjoyment in what we do is likely to encourage and promote learning of new skills and encourage the modification of existing ones. More 'natural' communication, based on more 'real' communicative needs is encouraged as part of therapy based on pragmatic principles (continued further in Chapter 7).

Whether one is engaged in communication because of a need or of being expected to do so, meanings that are expressed in either case can be intentional or unintentional (Levinson, 1983; also speech act theory, Chapter 3). When formulating a meaning expression the speaker intends it to be interpreted in a certain way by the listener: the speaker intends to express certain meanings rather than some others. Communication has taken place when the speaker's intention is recognized by the listener; communication is based on shared or mutual knowledge (Levinson, 1983). There are times, however, when the listener may attribute meanings to the expression that were not intended by the speaker. There are two primary cases where meanings can be unintentionally 'communicated'.

1. The listener reads into the expression meanings which are not present.
2. Meanings which the speaker did not intend to express are clearly manifest in the expression (perhaps non-verbally).

Meanings are communicated via listeners' minds, on the basis of their world knowledge and expectations, and as a consequence the received meaning may not correspond to the intended meaning. At times, the listener can be 'too creative' ('You are making all this up. I've said nothing like that'). Similarly, it is common for one to intend to express certain meanings, but unintentionally convey others. The meanings of language expressions are frequently modified and even overridden by non-verbal behaviours, paralinguistic cues and contextual variables. For instance, it is often fairly easy to tell that the speaker is not telling the truth by observing the shifts of gaze, fidgeting and other signs of discomfort. Saying 'I'd love to take part' with total lack of enthusiasm may imply 'I really don't want to be bothered with all this but if I have to I will'. When unintended meanings are being interpreted by a listener mutual communication has not taken place. While the notion of 'non-shared' communication is paradoxical in relation to the very definition of communication, and indeed poses problems for study of communication, the recognition of the existence of such unintentional meaning expression and interpretation has much clinical value. Indeed, communicative problems may stem from inability to match intention with expression, both in production and comprehension (Chapter 5). Furthermore, clinical appraisal of communication problems is likely to be affected by 'unintentional' expression and interpretation of meaning.

INTENTIONALITY AND CONVERSATIONAL PRINCIPLES

In addition to the intention to participate in interaction and the intention to express certain meanings over others, speakers intend meaning expressions, according to Grice (1975), to be informative, relevant, truthful and perspicuous. In other words, when communicating, speakers plan their expressions to have these overriding characteristics. And, when interpreting meanings, listeners operate on the principle that the speaker succeeds in his/her aim. Much of communication is based on this co-operative principle of the speaker having these overriding intentions and the listener believing that they underlie the speaker's meaning expressions. This idea constitutes Grice's Co-operative Principle which consists of four maxims.

1. The Maxim of Quantity: Speakers make their contributions as informative as required and not more or less informative than is required.
2. The Maxim of Quality: Speakers try not to say what they believe to be false or what lacks adequate evidence.
3. The Maxim of Relation: Speakers try to make contributions which are relevant.
4. The Maxim of Manner: Speakers try to avoid obscurity and ambiguity in meaning expression and try to be brief and orderly.

Both speakers and listeners are assumed to operate on the assumption that these principles are adhered to. They are conducive to smooth running of interaction by establishing some shared 'rules' upon which speakers and listeners rely. The operation of the maxims becomes apparent when they are flouted. Imagine the following exchange between two individuals.

A. I've been struggling with this nasty virus.
B. Oh, I'm sorry. Are you going to be all right?
A. I think I'll survive. The virus is in my computer.

While this example is somewhat artificial, it nevertheless neatly illustrates how flouting one of the maxims (that of Quantity) may lead to (momentary) misinterpretation of meaning. B's interpretation of A's utterance is inappropriate, because B assumes that A is giving the right amount of information, while clearly A is not giving enough information. The maxim of quality is also frequently flouted when language is used for the purpose of misleading. Similarly, meanings may not be communicated or may become hindered when the speaker's contributions seem not to be about the topic under discussion or are expressed in an obscure and ambiguous fashion ('When you ask him a question you never quite know whether he has answered it.'). This would constitute a violation of the maxim of relation. The maxim of manner is not adhered to when one seems not to know when to stop or when one jumps from one seemingly unrelated topic to another. The question is of course whether the maxims are violated purposely, as a means to an end, or are not adhered to because one is not aware of them or cannot implement them appropriately (pragmatic problem; Chapter 5). This kind of 'incoherent' language appears to be one of the defining characteristics of 'schizophrenic speech' (Rochester and Martin, 1979; Schwartz, 1982; Gordon, 1990).

Several other 'maxims' which govern and regulate communicative events can be identified. Leech (1983) discusses in some detail the Politeness Principle and its Maxims of Tact, Generosity, Approbation and Modesty. The Politeness Principle can be assumed to be operating in tandem with the Co-operative Principle by securing conversational participation and co-operation. Speakers tend to 'minimize (other things being equal) the expression of impolite beliefs' (p. 81) by minimizing cost to others (Tact Maxim), by minimizing benefit to self (Generosity Maxim), by maximizing praise of other (Approbation Maxim) and by minimizing praise of self (Modesty Maxim). Consider the following examples:

1. Could you lend me a pound? vs. Could I borrow a pound?
2. A: Your essay is very good.
   B: Yes, isn't it.

According to the maxims of Tact and Generosity, the second utterance in (1) is marginally more polite than the first in that it minimizes cost to the listener while maximizing cost to the speaker. In (2), A's utterance is motivated by the maxim of Approbation (compare 'Your essay is rather good'; 'Your essay is not too bad'), while B's utterance can be considered inappropriate by violating the maxim of Modesty. It could, of course, be a joke (and one hopes it was!; at least in the British culture).

The Politeness Principle has a relationship to the degree of directness in one's expression of meaning (see also Speech Act Theory, Chapter 3). Generally, the more indirect the expression, the more polite. This relationship is particularly culture bound. In some cultures, such as the Japanese, indirectness of expression and the degree of politeness are more closely related than in British English-speaking society. Similarly, within sub-cultures such as home, school and peer-group different degrees of politeness are appropriate. The case of irony presents an interesting dilemma: indicating a negative meaning by using polite conceptual meaning with 'an ironical' tone of voice ('That's great!') constitutes indeed a linguistically indirect expression of meaning, but from the point of view of societal politeness could be considered less polite than a more direct expression ('You should not have done that'). Politeness, as a principle of interpersonal communication, is explored in detail in Leech (1983) and Brown and Levinson (1978). Brown and Levinson draw particular attention to politeness as a face-saving device in communication.

Being aware of such principles which may govern communication provides some means of studying functioning and non-functioning individuals and communicative relationships. In the clinical context, one needs to be aware what one is aiming for in communication and how certain behaviours may indicate the absence of, or misinterpretation of such aims. As such, the notion of co-operation in communication provides an assessment framework for describing unsuccessful and successful communications (Chapters 4 and 6). Lack of adherence to the co-operative principles can also be indicative not only of lack of linguistic means for communicating, but, perhaps, of a pragmatically based problem (Chapter 5), of unhappiness, of anxiety or of a non-functioning communicative relationship. In particular, emphasizing the notion of co-operation, it highlights the need to consider not only what the client is doing or failing to do, but also how those interacting with the client might contribute toward the client's behaviour (Chapters 3 and 4). Communication is based on co-operation, and thus responsibility for both success and failure needs to be shared by all the participants (Chapters 4 and 6; also Leinonen and Smith, 1989). The co-operative aims also highlight some of the basic principles of pragmatically based therapy which focuses on facilitation of functional communication rather than linguistic accuracy (Chapter 7).

INTERIOR AND EXTERIOR COMMUNICATION

Studying communication most commonly refers to the study of overt communicative behaviours. In the clinical context we tend to focus on how the client expresses meanings and interacts when communicating with others. While this is obviously an important aspect to concentrate upon, what should not be forgotten is the centrality of the ability to 'communicate with oneself' for being able to share meanings with others.

We can distinguish between (i) communication within oneself (interior communication/dialogue/discourse; thinking; cognition) and (ii) communication with others (exterior communication/dialogue/discourse). The idea of communication within oneself can be somewhat paradoxical in that the term 'communication' by its very definition implies sharing of ideas, feelings, attitudes and other personal aspects of one's being. Can one share such things with oneself when they are in fact created within oneself? We can envisage an interior dialogue of questions and answers ('How do I really feel about being treated like this? I don't really like it. So, what am I going to do about it?' etc.) or other such mulling over of life's events. At one level, one could refer to this as sharing (communication) between one's conscious and sub-conscious selves. Whether such interior dialogue or discourse is strictly speaking 'communication' is not our main concern here. We simply want to emphasize the importance of one's ability to explain and evaluate life events and feelings to oneself and the importance of the ability to judge which thoughts and ideas are appropriate for sharing with others.

Our interior discourse can be thought of as forming the basis for shared communication. All communication is based on the ability to select and integrate – thoughts and events; past, present, future; words, phrases, sentences, utterances; gestures, facial expressions, gaze, movements; verbal expressions with non-verbal; our knowledge with our partners'. It is within oneself that these abilities evolve and unfold. Interior discourse is likely to share many features with the external expression of meanings, being based on the same cognitive premise of selection and integration. Yet, because of its non-interactive nature, it is likely to lack much of the explicitness and specificity of expression and linking required for sharing meanings. One can know what one means and how meanings link to form larger meaning networks without being able to put this knowledge into an overt expression. Most 'normally functioning' individuals can distinguish between interior and exterior discourse, can identify the central differences between them, can recognize the consequences of these differences for overt communication of meanings and can act upon this information. Those who have communication problems may have difficulty distinguishing between the two, and consequently their exterior discourse may resemble closely their less accessible interior discourse (Chapters 4 and 5). Those, for instance, who are diagnosed as suffering from mental disorders such as schizophrenia seem not to distinguish between interior and exterior discourse and consequently tend to produce overt expressions which others may find disjointed, incoherent, not specific enough, inappropriate, rude or idiosyncratic (e.g. Rochester and Martin, 1979; Schwartz, 1982; Chapter 5). Being able to monitor what to express overtly, and how, and what to keep to oneself is part of one's pragmatic competence (Chapter 5). Believing in the validity of one's own interior dialogue and view of the world is also important, but appears to be problematic for some disturbed children and adults (cf. Stott, 1966; temporal integration).

ASPECTS OF COMMUNICATION

In order to function as part of a society one needs to be able to share meanings with others. We shall now examine aspects of communication which can be considered central to one's ability to communicate. More specifically, we shall focus on those issues which we feel are of central importance to the clinical management of communication disorders. To keep this discussion manageable, we shall focus on dyadic (two-participant) interaction involving a speaker, a listener and a channel or medium of communication. The terms 'speaker' and 'listener' are used to refer to the more general notions of sender and receiver of messages.

The channel/medium

Starting with the channel/medium, it can be manifested orally/non-orally or verbally/non-verbally. Oral manifestations include expressions of meanings via the use of the oral mechanism for the production of sounds and noises; that is in:

1. Language realized in speech;
2. Interjections and fillers (e.g. 'tutting', 'um's and 'aah's);
3. Sighing, laughing, crying, singing;
4. Any other noises and vocalizations which have communicative value.

Non-oral expressions of meanings include:

1. Language manifested in writing;
2. Signing
3. Drawing
4. Gestures (audible and non-audible e.g. clapping, waving);
5. Facial expressions;
6. Gazing
7. Posture, proximics and other bodily orientations and movements with communicative value;
8. Communication aids.

The channel/medium of communication can also be manifested verbally or non-verbally. Verbal expressions of

meaning refer to signalling systems which have rule-
generatable structures and patterns. Thus, language manifested in speech or writing or sign language constitutes
verbal expressions of meaning. Non-verbal manifestations
of meaning include those orally produced noises which
are not organized into patterns and structures (e.g. interjections, fillers etc.) and those non-oral behaviours which
are customarily referred to as non-verbal behaviours in
communication (e.g. gestures of hands and arms, posture,
proximity, facial expressions, gaze etc.)

What is the significance of these distinctions to the practising clinician? Emphasis on communication via the oral
and verbal channels can easily become exaggerated, given
the centrality of language in human communication. In
the clinical contexts, emphasis tends to be on language
as manifested in speech, and to a lesser extent in writing
and signing. Focusing primarily on language as a medium
of communication can devalue the possibilities that other
means offer for communication. It is not uncommon to feel
somewhat surprised when one assesses the range of communicative functions and tasks clients with little or no access to language can perform by using other means. Many
have witnessed the delight of relatives and carers of such
individuals when made aware of the richness of communication that does, or can, take place, despite lack of
language. Being aware of handicapped individuals' capabilities can change one's perception of them as communicative partners and encourage one to interact and share
meanings more and at levels one did not feel were possible.

Non-oral and/or non-verbal means of communicating
can also provide a rich pool of devices for conveying complex and subtle meanings, to supplement and even replace verbal and oral expressions. Communication is about
being able to co-ordinate and combine different ways of
conveying meanings, via speech, writing, signing, gestures etc. and not merely about being able to produce well-
structured grammatical utterances with clear pronunciation
and unambiguous meaning. It is thus natural to encourage
multi-modal (using different channels simultaneously or
successively) communication with individuals with communication problems (Chapter 7). For instance, a mixture

of oral language and writing may be a workable means of communication for individuals who have difficulty in producing long stretches of language. The feasibility of the expression of meanings via different channels is dependent on many factors. The nature and severity of the client's handicap constrain and restrict the choices available. The communicative purpose is also an influencing factor. The breadth and depth of meanings, which can be expressed via means other than language, can be limited and thus at times such expressions may have limited communicative use. It is equally important to consider what the listener is capable of processing. A trained speech-language professional may be much more skilled in interpreting and processing meaning signals than a person with no training in behavioural observation. Similarly, those familiar with the client, such as partners, friends, parents, siblings and teachers, are likely to find communicating with the client easier than those unfamiliar with him/her. There are various influences outside the client bearing upon the channel via which communication is possible. These outside influences can also be worked with to enhance and encourage successful communication. Educating those who interact with communicatively handicapped individuals to consider and accommodate specific individual problems has always been (to varying degrees) part of the management of disability.

The distinctions between oral/non-oral and verbal/nonverbal gain added relevance in the clinical management of communication disorders if an attempt is made to correlate these distinctions with types of disorders. The correlation can be based on the potential of the individual with a communication disorder to use the oral/non-oral or verbal/nonverbal means for expressing meanings. Such correlation can lead to suggestions for possible ways of expressing meanings. A severely apraxic person may be considered primarily as being able to use the verbal/non-oral channels for communication (non-oral with the reservation that most people have some oral capacity for producing vocalizations and/or sounds, which in turn may have communicative value). This 'classification' may then lead to suggestions for possible means of communication. In this case, verbal or non-verbal expressions of meanings which are not orally manifested (e.g. signing, gesturing, writing, drawing). Or, we may be dealing with a client suffering from a severe head injury. He or she might be considered oral and non-verbal. Possible means of communicating include non-patterned (i.e. non-verbal) oral or non-oral means (e.g. vocalizations, gestures, drawing). While this kind of correlational exercise is in many ways artificial in that it doesn't fully appreciate the multi-faceted nature of various types of disorders, it nevertheless gives some justifiable guidelines for attempting to broaden the communicative experience of those who may miss out on interacting with others because of their particular handicaps. In actual clinical practice, the artificiality of such an approach is diminished by experienced clinicians who are capable of making informed decisions concerning the client's capabilities. Indeed, such a correlational exercise is only a means of clarifying for the benefit of future clinicians what the practising clinician does intuitively.

Precursors for the formulation, expression and interpretation of meanings

To be able to express and interpret meanings in communicative encounters, there are certain prerequisite skills and abilities the speaker and listener need to possess. Communication is possible without some of these skills and the extent of use of them can vary considerably from individual to individual and in different communicative contexts. Compensatory strategies may also be employed by the interactants to alleviate or overcome lack of the prerequisites. The following discussion is by no means exhaustive: the purpose of this section is simply to outline what can be considered as the main prerequisite abilities for communication to be possible at all.

To be able to manipulate signs and signals for expressing meanings in communication, it is necessary to hold and relate events and experiences in one's mind. This **cognitive ability** is a basic prerequisite, given that communication is based on selection and integration of knowledge, which needs to be held in both long-term and working memory.

The ability to attend to tasks, to relate cause and effect and to appreciate object permanence are other important cognitive prerequisites. Similarly, all forms of communication require some **motor ability**, however minimal. When articulating sounds, signing, writing, gesturing, gazing etc., various types of motor movements need to be controlled and co-ordinated. Equally, communication is dependent on **perceptual ability**. Cognitive resources, experiences and knowledge of the world are shaped by perceptual experiences. What we see, hear, feel and taste forms the basis of what we know, and thus can communicate about. It is our cognitive resources which link and join these perceptual experiences into meanings, and it is probably then our emotions and aesthetic sense which endow these meanings with significance and relative importance or unimportance.

When engaged in the 'here-and-now' of a communicative encounter cognitive and perceptual abilities are called upon in deciding which meanings have been expressed previously in the encounter, and thus what can be expressed next in order for the next contribution to be relevant to the ongoing discourse. Cognitive abilities also enable us to presuppose what our communicative partner knows about the world around us, and thus what can be assumed known, and left unexpressed and what is likely to be regarded as relevant and interesting. Observing our immediate environment, the objects, people and behaviours which characterize it, also influences the formulation, expression and interpretation of meanings. For instance, in conversational encounters, as speakers we closely observe, more or less successfully, the verbal and non-verbal signals of understanding/not understanding, interest/boredom, anger/ joy and so on given by our partners, and this observation creates, directs and constrains what we express and how.

If the medium of communication is that of language, spoken or written, in addition to the above kinds of general abilities, the speaker and listener require 'language ability'. (There are various prerequisites for the development of language ability, the discussion of which is beyond the scope of the present book.) For the present purposes, this ability can be thought of as separate from the motor ability to articulate sounds and the ability to use language in communication (e.g. Curtiss, 1988). This 'ability' can be thought of as equalling the knowledge of language structures consisting of the knowledge of:

1. How sounds can be combined to form words according to the conventions of the ambient language;
2. The nature and function of tone, rhythm, pitch, stress and intonation patterns;
3. How words can be combined to form sentences/ utterances;
4. How sentences/utterances can be combined to form longer stretches of text;
5. Meanings interrelated with real life referents and concepts.

The aspects of language structure specified in (1) are studied within the linguistic fields of phonology (segmental) and morphology; those specified in (2) within suprasegmental phonology; those specified in (3) within syntax, those specified in (4) within discourse analysis or text linguistics; and those specified in (5) within semantics. The assumption is that language exists independently of meanings created within individuals and in communicative contexts. In other words, we cannot even begin to express meanings in communication via language unless we possess decontextualized knowledge of language.

Is it reasonable to assume that language exists in such decontextualized terms? Autistic children are said to 'have language' but have problems in using it in communication (e.g. Rutter, 1978). Structures and patterns of the ambient language can be relatively easily identified in their language output, yet it may make little, if any, sense. Similarly, many in the English speaking world are familiar with Lewis Carroll's famous poem 'Jabberwocky' where 'Twas brillig and the slithey toves. Did gyre and gimble in the wabe', where sounds combine into words without conventional meaning. Similarly, sentences can have recognizable structure without interpretation: those familiar with Chomsky (1965) cannot forget how 'Colourless green ideas sleep furiously' – the famous meaningless sentence with an identifiable grammatical structure. We can also identify longer stretches of sentences and utterances as having coherence and structure of texts without understanding their (full) meaning. At one extreme, we can recognize a conversation between individuals using a language we are not familiar with. Or, we can easily produce a non-sensical text (e.g. using connecting words and expressions such as 'however', 'therefore', 'as was indicated above' etc.). Such discourse structures are identifiable, for instance, in the language of schizophrenic patients, even though the overall message of the discourse may be unreachable (e.g. Rochester and Martin, 1979; Gordon, 1990). Decontextualized word meanings can also be thought of as existing. These are the 'core', 'conceptual' or 'dictionary' meanings of words and idiomatic phrases (Lyons, 1977). The word 'dog', as most people would agree, refers to a furry animal, kept as a pet by humans. There are certain 'dogginess' characteristics which define the commonly 'shared' (i.e. core, conceptual, dictionary) meaning of this word. For communication to be possible via language such shared meanings need to exist. But these core meanings are moulded by individuals and communicative contexts. 'Dog' to one person may mean 'a lovable pet' and to another 'a barking, fouling creature next door'. Similarly, 'She's a real dog' referring to a woman has a sexist meaning rather different from the core meaning. In these instances the decontextualized meaning of the word 'dog' has beome context-specific.

This decontextualized pool of language structures, the language knowledge (also referred to as language competence or language system, Chapters 2, 4 and 5), forms the resource we make choices from in communication. Similarly, we can envisage a pool of non-verbal expressions which can be used for communication.

Making choices is likely to be largely unconscious, yet there are occasions when 'choosing one's words (expression) carefully' can be a very conscious exercise. For those who tend to make inappropriate choices from the pool of not only language expressions but meaning expressions in general, it may be necessary to bring into consciousness the influences and motivations for the particular choices. The influences which make us choose one expression over another range from the above kinds of cognitive, perceptual and motor constraints to numerous social, contextual, cultural and other such motivations.

Influences bearing upon meaning formulation, expression and interpretation

Given that cognitive, perceptual, motor and language abilities affect our ability to express and interpret meanings appropriately, there are also various other influences which shape the communicative event. Which meanings are expressed and how depends on factors such as:

1. The meanings that have been expressed previously;
2. The nature of the communicative context;
3. The communicative partner and relationship;
4. The purpose of communication;
5. Personality characteristics including the creativity of the speaker;
6. The speaker's educational and cultural background.

Let us consider each of these factors in turn to illustrate their potential roles in communication.

1. The meanings which have been previously expressed regulate the relevance of the present utterance to the ongoing topic. Previous discourse can constrain both the content and the form of utterances. People are expected to talk about the topics under discussion and to be able to do so one needs not only to understand what has been expressed previously but also to find the topics sufficiently interesting to merit further comment. It is of course appropriate to change the topic and there are devices for topical change and shift (Chapter 3) which render talking about a different topic from the immediately previous relevant and appropriate ('I know that this is not directly related to what you have just said, but . . .'). Knowing when it is appropriate to shift or change the focus of discussion and how to do so appropriately is part of one's pragmatic competence (Chapters 2 and 5). What has gone before can also determine the words, and even the grammatical structures used. 'I agree with that' is appropriate only if we can determine from the previous utterances what 'that' refers to (Chapter 3).

2. The physical environment in which the communicative event takes place can affect the relevance and the informativeness of the meaning expressions. 'I want that one' accompanied by pointing is only relevant and informative if there are appropriate referents in the context to which 'that' can refer. In this way, the perceptibility of referents in the communicative context can restrict the content and form of the expression. The physical environment also affects the channel via which communication is possible. Signing, gesturing or mouthing may be the only means available for attempting to convey meanings when communicating through a barrier such as a window. Communicative contexts can also vary according to their formality and other characteristics and communicative expectations. Different communicative behaviours are manifested during Prime Minister's Question Time (a mixture of communicative behaviours which are probably only acceptable in this particular context), a board meeting, speech therapy sessions carried out in a clinic or at the client's home, a party held at the office or on the beach and so on.

3. Similarly, who our communicative partner is shapes the content and the form of meaning expressions. The status, age, sex, cultural and educational background, race and any other social variable concerning the communicative partner contribute towards choosing expressions which are more or less polite, honest, spontaneous, risky, interesting and so on. Different surface expressions conveying the same conceptual meanings feel appropriate when interacting with males or females, with people we perceive as higher or lower status in relation to ourselves, with people of different generations, with people with whom we are familiar or with strangers and so on. The appropriateness of these utterances is also constrained by the communicative purpose of the interaction: we may want to offend or be polite. The speaker's perception of the ability of the communicative partner to process meaning expressions also affects what is expressed and how. Talking to children, foreigners, handicapped individuals and the elderly induces language simplified in structure and content and increased in repetition. Informativeness, relevance, brevity and politeness may suffer as a consequence. Simi-

larly, the speaker needs to be able to assess what the communicative partner knows about the world: that is, what their life experiences are likely to be, thus affecting their knowledge of different topic areas and their spheres of interest. Stating the obvious or talking well above somebody's head are problems encountered in many conversational interactions. Formulation and expression of meanings are also constrained by the type of feedback the listener gives the speaker, or has given during previous encounters. The verbal and non-verbal cues dispensed by the 'active' listener in the form of back channel responses (minimal responses) may make speakers feel relaxed or hurried, enthusiastic or reluctant, affecting the expression of meanings accordingly.

4. Meaning expressions have a purpose to them. Speakers may wish to inform, question, direct other people's behaviour, make a good impression, offend, joke, chat up, put off and perform other acts beyond simply stating the existence of concepts and objects (Speech act theory, Chapter 3). Much of communication is motivated by personal needs which can be satisfied by communicating with others (see intention, above). It is the underlying personal needs which may motivate us to engage in communication in the first instance, or may make us withdraw and which may motivate us to aim for one communicative goal rather than another (Communication strategies; Chapter 3). Communication is goal-oriented behaviour and its manifestation is created and constrained by the specific goals.

5. Personality, creativity, imaginativeness and other such personal characteristics also shape what one communicates about and how one goes about it. Being outgoing or reserved, more or less creative and so on determines the communicative style of the individual, influencing the length of contributions, the content of utterances and, overall, whether one's personal and communicative goals are likely to be realized. Since communication is often an uncertain business of not knowing how one's meanings will be received and an activity on the basis of which others form expressions about oneself, those who are risk-takers and less concerned about portraying a particular image are more likely to achieve their goals. It is not difficult to see how personality characteristics of those with communica-

tive handicaps can have a powerful influence on how problems are coped with: there may be those who attempt to communicate with whatever means are available in order not to become socially isolated, potentially compromising communicative efficiency and exposing one's handicap. There are also those who may feel unable to show weakness, thus avoiding situations in which one's problems may become exposed, and thus potentially compromising personal and communicative goals.

6. Rules and behaviour patterns imposed by cultures and sub-cultures also influence communicative encounters. Directness of expression, degree of politeness, gestures and proximics are largely culturally bound. Being part of a family, being a student, a single parent, a golfer or a railway enthusiast influences our interaction within the particular social groups and outside them. Our life experiences provide us with conversational topics, specialized vocabulary and a particular slant on life. Our educational background is also a powerful influencing factor on how we interact with others: it provides knowledge, and social skills, which in turn may promote or belittle one's 'communicative self-esteem'.

Throughout this discussion emphasis has been on the speaker, on the influences which bear upon the formulation and expression of meanings. Very much the same influences affect the interpretation of meanings (McGregor, 1986). The listener's comprehension of meanings is influenced by his:

1. Ability to select and integrate events and experiences in mind;
2. Ability to perceive auditory, visual and other perceptual signals;
3. Ability to attend;
4. Ability to process verbal and non-verbal meaning expressions;
5. Cultural and educational background;
6. Personality characteristics including creativity and imaginativeness;
7. Relationship with the speaker, including familiarity, shared interests and degree of empathy;

8. Purpose in participating in the interaction;
9. Processing of what has been expressed before;
10. The cognitive complexity of the topic under discussion (Brown, 1989).

There are numerous factors which make us interpret similar messages in different ways and different messages in similar ways. Listeners not only use overt expressions as guidelines to interpretation but engage in active creation of meanings, using their knowledge of the world, of the communicative context, of purpose, of participants and of human interaction in general as a basis for inferencing. We shall not discuss interpretation of meanings in much detail in the current volume, simply because of our lack of expertise in the area. Yet, because of its centrality in the communication process, we wish not to ignore it, and will therefore discuss 'the listener' wherever appropriate, albeit not exhaustively.

Reciprocity in communication

It does not suffice to be able to express and interpret meanings appropriately: we need to know when to stop talking and yield the floor and when to stop listening and take the floor. Communication is essentially reciprocal: somebody expresses a meaning and somebody else responds. As such communication is basically a sequence of initiations and responses (Exchange structure, Chapter 3). Part of one's communicative ability is to be aware of this basic structure of communication and to be able to judge in real communicative encounters when it is appropriate to make one's contribution and when it is appropriate to listen to others. This judgment in turn is dependent on one's ability to understand what has been said previously, to formulate a relevant contribution, to ascertain how turns at speaking and listening are allocated and to determine when the previous speaker has come to an end of a turn, thus potentially offering the floor to someone else. This constitutes knowledge of turn-taking dynamics, which are discussed in detail in Chapter 3.

SUMMARY

We have now outlined what communication generally involves from the speakers' and listeners' perspective. There
are certain prerequisite skills, abilities and other factors
which shape communicative behaviour. Meaning expressions, including language expressions, are created, constrained and restricted by these abilities and factors. While
the discussion of these issues here is necessarily superficial,
given the breadth and depth of influences bearing upon
communication, it nevertheless serves a purpose of as-
sembling the main features together in one place. In this
way, we can capture the interrelatedness and interaction
of factors shaping human communication, thus attempting to dispense with the artificiality of approaches which
study human communication in terms of separate skills
and abilities (Chapters 2 and 4).

Chapter 2

Pragmatics, discourse analysis and clinical pragmatics

Having discussed many of the factors involved in communication in Chapter 1, we can now examine how the study of pragmatics and discourse fits into this discussion.

PRAGMATICS

Probably the earliest interest in the use of language and the influences which bear upon it was displayed by ancient orators in speech making and debating. Ancient rhetoric was concerned with the means by which speeches produce a desired effect on the audience. It was concerned with construction of logical arguments and other such communicative behaviours involving effective use of language. In modern terms, these enterprises involve pragmatic considerations of matching linguistic expressions with contextual considerations: What is the nature of the audience? What is the purpose of the speech? (Chapter 1). Speech making and debating also involve linking of utterances and the development of topics and arguments. These can be studied as a function of coherence relationships and cohesive links within the modern paradigm of discourse analysis (Discourse analysis, below; also Chapter 3).

While such early philosophical approaches constitute a foundation for the study of language use, the field of pragmatics, as we know it today, can be envisaged as having primarily evolved from:

1. Semiotic study of signs and their meanings (Peirce, 1960, Barthes, 1968, Eco, 1976);

2. Twentieth-century philosophical approaches to language (Morris, 1938, Austin, 1962, Searle, 1969);
3. Linguistic investigations of functional aspects of language expressions (Firth, 1957, Halliday, 1967, 1973, Danes, 1974).

Semiotics and pragmatics

Semiotics, the study of how signs and symbols have meaning, is the all-encompassing study of communication. It is concerned with all human symbolic systems, be they language, gestures, pictures, films or road signs. As such, semiotics is concerned with 'meanings and messages in all their forms and in all their contexts' (Innis, 1985, vii). In its quest for a general theory of signs, semiotics attempts to define what a sign is, why signs exist at all, how different types of signs stand in relation to one another in a system of signs, what powers signs have and so on. Being dynamic, evolving entities, signs are studied within the communication process. Signs gain meaning within the human mind and human communication and thus meanings are created on the basis of cognitive, psychological, sociological, cultural, contextual and interactional influences (Chapter 1).

Defined as such, we can locate other specific fields of enquiry into human communication within the study of semiotics. For instance, the various sub-fields of linguistics, by considering the sign system of language, constitute a study of applied semiotics. Linguistics 'proper' (excluding applied fields) develops the theory and description of the sign system of language. Similarly, various areas of psychology contribute towards the understanding of signs and meaning creation, and in particular towards understanding their role in creating human knowledge in general. As such psychological investigations can be considered within the umbrella of semiotics. The same can be said to be true of sociology, ethnomethodology and anthropology which investigate meanings as part of societies, interactions and cultures.

How does the study of pragmatics fit into this conception of semiotics? Pragmatics can be defined as the study of how expressions of meaning by humans gain significance in context and use (see further below). This stems from the ideas of early philosophical and political pragmatists who believed that humans have choices with regard to making communication work or not work and that these choices can be studied separately from the communicative systems within which they are made. In this way, it is the study of pragmatics which examines how meaning expressions come into being and which influences bear upon their formulation, expression and interpretation (Chapter 1). It examines how humans make choices from the signalling systems available and how these choices shape the communicative event. Defined as such, pragmatics is a branch of semiotics, but having a narrower focus. Pragmatics investigates only human signalling systems while all sign systems constitute the domain of study for semiotics.

Philosophical influences on pragmatics

Notwithstanding the centrality of semiotic notions for the development of the study of human communication in general, and the field of pragmatics in particular, semiotics has not however provided any theory or methodology for these fields. This is simply a reflection of the absence of pure semiotic study. Modern philosophers (Morris, 1938, Austin, 1962, Searle, 1969; also Wittgenstein, 1958), however, have had a greater influence on how the field of pragmatics is perceived and studied.

Morris (1938) defined pragmatics as the study of 'the relation of signs to interpreters' (p. 6). In examining this relationship, the study of psychological, sociological, neurological, cultural and any other relevant influences bearing upon signs and signification was considered within pragmatic study. This is a much wider approach to language usage than that adopted by modern (linguistic) pragmatics (Levinson, 1983, Leech, 1983, Sperber and Wilson, 1986). Its breadth however is of crucial importance when applied to the study of communication disorders (Clinical pragmatics below; also Chapter 4). While Morris's ideas have been influential in the development of 'the science of pragmatics' (see below), it is Austin's (1962) speech act theory (Chapter 3) which has had the most appreciable effect on what now constitutes study matter for pragmatics. Austin was interested in how utterances have both conceptual meaning and communicative force, which signals the intention underlying the utterance. By producing language people can make promises, insult others, invite or avoid conflict, tell jokes, manipulate others; in other words, language expressions carry meaning beyond the literal meanings of the co-occurring words. The functions that utterances have in different context and communicative encounters is one of the central concerns of modern pragmatics and functional linguistics.

The study of deictic expressions and presupposition within the pragmatic paradigm also derives from philosophical tradition. This involves the study of how deictic expressions (or indexicals) such as 'She is unhappy' gain meaning for the listener via association of the word 'she' with the real life referent. When producing a deictic expression the speaker needs to presuppose appropriately whether it is possible for the listener to recover the referent, and thus the meaning, of the deictic form (i.e. 'she'). The notion of presupposition which constitutes a vast area of study within pragmatics (Levinson, 1983), derives from logical semantics (e.g. Strawson, 1952, Keenan, 1971) and from its concern for semantic inferences or presuppositions when determining truth values and truth conditions of sentences (Lyons, 1977, Levinson, 1983). From semantic inference, the notion of pragmatic inference or presupposition developed to consider the contextual meanings of utterances. Another kind of pragmatic inference, which constitutes an area of study within pragmatics, was also developed by a philosopher. Grice's (1975, 1978) conversational implicatures and conversational principles address the activity of inferencing as a co-operative enterprise of meaning negotiation (Chapter 1).

Linguistics and pragmatics

Much of the current literature on pragmatics deals exclusively with linguistic pragmatics. Linguistic pragmatics concentrates on the language expression, rather than on expression of meanings via other means (e.g. non-verbal;

proximics), and constitutes consequently a narrower conception of the field than was envisaged by philosophers such as Morris (1938) and by the study of clinical pragmatics as explored in the current volume. Indeed, pragmatics is commonly defined in relation to the linguistic field of semantics as 'meaning minus semantics' (Levinson, 1983, 31). According to this, pragmatics studies those aspects of meaning in language which semantics does not address. While in theory this conceptualization of the study matter for pragmatics seems a fairly workable one, determining the boundaries between semantic and pragmatic study of meaning is problematic (Levinson, 1983). In very broad terms, pragmatics can be regarded as a study of contextual meaning and semantics the study of decontextual meaning (Lyons, 1977, Levinson, 1983). To illustrate this distinction consider the following:

Decontextual meanings	*Possible contextual meanings*
'Charming' = delightful	'Charming!' = not very nice
'You shouldn't have' = ought not to have done	'You shouldn't have' = what a lovely present
'Is that personal toast?' = Does that toast belong to you?	'Is that personal toast?' = Could I have that toast?

Linguistic pragmatics is interested in contextually created meaning. In communication, all meanings are contextual by virtue of gaining significance in contexts, in people's minds and through people's experiences. Yet, despite differences in life experiences, many meaning expressions in similar cultures are interpreted in similar ways. These shared meanings constitute the 'semantic storehouse' of meanings, the decontextual meanings, which then become contextualized via human experience and interaction.

Formal and functional approaches to language

Historically, linguistics and pragmatics have been worlds apart. The study of linguistics 'proper' had for many years concentrated on language structure alone without much regard for language use. This concentration on the formal linguistic structures alone has been referred to as the formal paradigm (Dik, 1978). In formal descriptions of language structure no note is taken of the feasibility of structures in human communication, of their meanings or acceptability in communicative contexts. It was widely maintained that the study of language structure has logical priority over the study of the use of structures for communicative ends (e.g. Bloomfield, 1933; Chomsky, 1965; see also Radford, 1988). It was argued that one cannot begin to study how structures are used in communication or how structures are acquired in language development if one doesn't first know what the structures themselves are. While this is clearly a convincing argument, the formal approaches to language (such as the Transformational Generative Grammar, Chomsky, 1965) were criticized for being too non-motivated by human communication. The structural frameworks devised produced sentences which were too complex or long to be handled by human information-processing capacity at any given time and which did not provide information about contexts in which sentences could or could not be used. Such structuralist approaches also considered human language as being made of components; as a complex network of larger components which consist of smaller components. Thus, sentences are perceived as being made of clauses, clauses of phrases, phrases of words, words of morphemes, morphemes of phonemes and phonemes of features.

A formal approach to language, as briefly outlined above, is only valid if it serves the purpose it was devised to serve. The main aims of such structuralist approaches were to describe particular languages in order to describe language universals (i.e. features which all human languages have in common) and to describe the knowledge native speakers of language have about the structure of language (Chomsky's notion of competence, Chapter 5). Because language is productive in that novel utterances can be produced and comprehended by people, the speakers and listeners are likely to operate with linguistic rules. Also, the aim of formal approaches was to describe the rules which characterize specific linguistic systems. Contextual influences shaping human communication are not the domain of such linguistic descriptions.

Accepting that each area of study is entitled to define its domain and keep within its aims and constraints, the formal approach has, nevertheless, been the subject of much controversy. It has been questioned whether it serves any purpose to divorce the knowledge of language structure and its description from its use (Interaction of linguistic levels, Chapter 4). In other words, the knowledge of structure is likely to be intrinsically interwoven with, and motivated by, the knowledge of language use (Levinson, 1983; linguistic competence vs. communicative competence, Chapter 5). Thus, it has been suggested that exploring linguistic knowledge and the nature of universals in the context of language use may be more meaningful for understanding human communication as a whole, and the place of linguistic structure within this whole. Within this premise, functional approaches to linguistic structure emerged.

Alongside the structuralist schools of, notably, Bloomfield and Chomsky, less influential (at that point) proponents of a functional approach to language existed. Writers such as Firth in the 1930 to 1950s (Firth, 1957) and Halliday from the 1960s onwards (e.g. Halliday, 1967, 1973) developed taxonomies for studying language structure in terms of its function in communication. Concurrently, the Prague School of Linguistics developed the Functional Sentence Perspective approach to explore the role of the sentence in text in terms of its organization as information (Danes, 1974; Coherence, Informativity, Chapter 3). All these approaches considered contextual influences as integral aspects of the theory of language structure. A strong school of functional linguistics has since developed which draws upon, and feeds into, the study of pragmatics (Dik, 1978, Halliday, 1985). In the functional approach, language is considered as a vehicle of social interaction and linguistic description is considered valid if it manages to capture what influences language choices in use and how language use influences language structure. With the development of functional linguistics and the various fields of applied linguistics, exploring social (sociolinguistics), psychological (psycholinguistics) and other influences shaping communication, the overlap between linguistics and pragmatics is considerable. It does not particularly matter whether these areas of enquiry constitute separate disciplines or one being inclusive of another. What matters, however, is the recognition that the study of human communication is an interdisciplinary enterprise and ventures well beyond the study of language structure, or even language function, into the study of (almost) everything that shapes and moulds communication into what it is when it happens in real contexts.

Principles from both formal and functional approaches to language have been applied to the study and management of language pathology. For the past twenty years or so (Relevance, below), speech pathology in certain contexts (notably those of child language and stroke rehabilitation) has focused a great deal on formal linguistic structures and systems, studying and assessing these fairly separately from language use. Language disability is often studied in terms of phonological, syntactic and semantic systems with perhaps minimal, if any, regard for the interrelatedness of these systems (Interaction of linguistic levels, Chapter 4). Language is considered a collection of components rather than an integrated whole. The implications of this for assessment, diagnosis and management, and consequently for one's perception of the client's abilities and disabilities, are far-reaching (Chapters 4, 5, 6 and 7). While it cannot be disputed that to be able to communicate via language one requires knowledge about the structure of language, it does not follow that knowledge of this structure is necessarily accessible and assessible or that acquisition of such knowledge guarantees its use. It is essential to explore such issues in the clinical context in order to work on aspects of language and communication which are psychologically real and socially useful for the client.

Pragmatics: main areas of study

Pragmatics focuses on many aspects of communication, both from the producer's and the receiver's perspectives. This is not however to suggest that all the various fields of study which address communicative phenomena (e.g. linguistics, anthropology, social psychology etc.) constitute a sub-field within pragmatics. Nor that pragmatics does not constitute a study in its own right. The field of pragmatics can be perceived as having two functions. Firstly, it studies certain communicative phenomena which other fields of enquiry do not address in the same fashion. Secondly, being concerned with human communication in the widest sense of the term it focuses on the interrelatedness of the various other fields of inquiry. As such, the study of pragmatics provides a forum within which the various disciplines can be brought together to examine human communication in its entirety.

Keeping in mind the difficulties in defining pragmatics as a study of contextual meaning, certain areas of inquiry can however be attributed to the field of pragmatics. Broadly speaking, pragmatics aims to specify conditions for speakers choosing a particular meaning expression over others and for listeners interpreting meanings in certain ways rather than in others. Within this premise, the study of pragmatics addresses the following main issues (see also Levinson, 1983)

1. **intentionality** underlying meaning expressions (Chapter 1). What did the speaker intend the meaning expression to convey? Intentionality is primarily studied in terms of the notion of speech acts (or communicative acts; Chapter 3); in terms of what speakers aim to achieve in communication and whether they do so and in terms of how intention is reflected in the meaning expression itself. Listeners' perception of speaker intention is also of interest, despite the inherent difficulties in studying the effect expressed intention may have on the listener.
2. **conversational principles or implicatures** such as Grice's (Chapter 1). Their role in governing co-operation in communication and negotiation of meanings between participants is a major area of interest within pragmatics.
3. **presupposition** in terms of what meaning expressions themselves presuppose or entail and of what the speakers and listeners need to be able to presuppose for communication to be successful (e.g. presuppose what the other person knows) (Chapter 3). Considering how the

interpretation of meaning expressions (e.g. deictic items) is context-dependent is part of this inquiry.

4. **how communication is 'managed'**. This involves examination of metacommunicative behaviours, of who controls the flow of communication and of the extent of shared responsibility.
5. **the appropriateness** of meaning expressions: in which contexts and why speakers and listeners find communicative behaviours appropriate or inappropriate (Chapter 4).
6. **the choices** speakers and listeners have and **the constraints** which are placed upon meaning expression and interpretation in social interaction.

When studying communicative phenomena within a pragmatic framework, the focus is on processes by which the specific communicative behaviours come into being rather than the behavioural product (Leech, 1983). Process-oriented approaches to meaning creation in communication are of particular value in the clinical context. Exploring how successful and unsuccessful communicative encounters and/or appropriate or inappropriate communicative behaviours came into being enables one to identify communicative strengths and potential sources of difficulty which in turn feed into well-motivated management methods and strategies (Clinical pragmatics, below; also, Chapter 4). Such methods and strategies are well-motivated since they are based on aspects of communication which are socially and psychologically valid for the client.

Science of pragmatics?

Communication is a subjective experience by its very nature. Meanings are created in people's minds and no two minds are alike. Does this render the study of communication, and pragmatics in particular, a haphazard and 'non-scientific' activity and one not worth pursuing too seriously? Whether pragmatics constitues a 'proper' science has been a subject of many discussions and their general 'conclusions' are worth reiterating here in order to clarify any misconceptions which might exist.

'A scientific paradigm' as applied to the study of human communication appears to promote two fallacies. The first is that communicative phenomena (or, in fact, any phenomena) can be observed objectively. That is to say that there is some absolute 'truth' which is constant and unnegotiable in human existence. The second is that communicative phenomena can be described in terms of precise rules.

The first of these is a fallacy since all observation is through the eyes, the ears, mind, capabilities and experiences of the observer, and thus involves interpretation. While the same phenomenon can be, and often is, interpreted in a similar fashion, identical interpretation of a phenomenon is a near impossibility since it assumes identical life experiences, perceptual experiences and so on. Similarity of observation and interpretation is however promoted by our common experiences in similar cultures and sub-cultures and by the very fact that we are all human. People are also trained in observational techniques which promote uniformity (=objectivity) of interpretation. Phonemic transcription of a client's speech is an example of such a technique. Given this argument, promoting objectivity in the observation of behaviour means promoting similarity of observation and interpretation by diminishing intersubject variability. While communication is a personal experience, there is much agreement as to what is appropriate or inappropriate in any particular culture. Promoting awareness of what constitutes communication, of the influences which shape it (Chapter 1), promotes heightened awareness of what communication entails and of its fluid and changeable nature. The study of pragmatics is interested in a descriptive, not prescriptive, approach to discovering principles which motivate language use in human communication.

Secondly, the non-scientific reputation of the study of pragmatics is founded in its historical role as a 'dustbin' for those communicative phenomena which cannot be described in terms of precise rules. Linguistic description of language, being interested in rules which generate language structures, had to discard those contextual or pragmatic aspects of communication which were too complex and variable to lend themselves to rules (the Chomskian era; Chomsky, 1965, Radford, 1988). Being scientific in the linguistic sense was then equated with language being describable in terms of context-independent rules. In more recent years, functional grammars (Dik, 1978, Halliday, 1985) have attempted to write rules to account for variability in communication. Language use, being affected by so many factors, is difficult to describe in terms of rules and thus, more often than not, several exceptions to a rule can be found. Approaches to 'pragmatic' phenomena, such as speech act theory and the study of presuppositions, have also attempted to outline context-sensitive rules or conditions for language use (e.g. Searle, 1969, Levinson, 1983). These would specify, for instance, the conditions under which one could make a promise and under which it would come off as one. Such principles attempt to capture the general conditions for language use and obviously cannot account for specific instances (e.g. the conditions underlying promises made by lovers can vary greatly from those made by enemies). Writing a separate rule for every occurrence of language use would defy the whole purpose of rules. Conditions or principles underlying communicative use of language, or any signalling of meanings, are variable, yet the fact that such principles can be identified signifies that 'not anything goes'. Being 'scientific, methodological and systematic, in one's approach to communication, does not necessitate description of communicative phenomena in terms of non-variable rules since communication itself varies in different contexts. A pragmatic approach attempts to specify these variable conditions for communication, recognizing that there is no absolute norm, no absolute right or wrong, and thus the conditions are general ones, subject to further contextual modification.

The issue of whether a science of pragmatics can exist and what the nature of this would be was discussed by a panel of distinguished proponents of the pragmatic approach in the 2nd Meeting of the International Pragmatics Association in 1987 (Verschueren, 1987). The panel concluded that ultimately it doesn't really matter whether pragmatics can be called a science or not: communicative phenomena are real and interesting enough to warrant serious study and investigation, and analytical methods and principles for studying the phenomena in a systematic manner exist. It was however felt that pragmatics having the status of a science could have a unifying influence on a field of study which in its present form is still young and insecure and which covers a wide and diverse area of interests. In defence of pragmatics as a non-scientific contextual dustbin, Mey, in the above panel, observed that 'of course they [theories of grammar like the Transformational Generative Grammar of Chomsky, 1965] can be successful, because you define the work that you have to do yourself. Then, of course, you can be very successful at that. But it doesn't mean that your theory is good because you do a piece of work which you have sort of carved out for yourself' (Verschueren, 1987; 38–39) (cf. formal vs. functional approaches above). In the clinical context, the communicative behaviours of clients are not ignored simply because they cannot be neatly described. In a clinical pragmatic approach, the 'carving out' of the task will be minimized, and phenomena will not be left unaccounted for simply because they do not fit into a particular framework of study (below, and Chapter 4).

DISCOURSE AND DISCOURSE ANALYSIS

The same communicative language phenomena can be studied both within the field of pragmatics and that of discourse analysis. Initiation/response sequences, Grice's communicative principles, speech acts and deictic expressions are some of the main areas of inquiry covered in both disciplines. Is there any difference and thus a need for the two disciplines? Let us begin exploring this question by considering how the terms discourse and discourse analysis are generally perceived in the literature.

Beyond the everyday use of the term discourse to refer to conversation and dialogue, it has also more theoretical foundations and meanings. The meaning of discourse in the academic study of discourse analysis derives from the dichotomy of formal and functional approaches to language (as above). A single, isolated sentence was the object of study of formal grammars ('sentence grammars'). No note was taken of the occurrence of sentences in communicative contexts and in real time. In other words, no note was taken of the social and cognitive influences which bear upon language when used in communication. The real forms of language use, reflecting such influences, were termed discourse. Thus, reference is made to different discourse types or genres reflecting language use in different contexts (e.g. informal discourse, formal discourse, legal discourse, caregiver-child discourse, therapeutic discourse and narrative discourse). Discourse analysis is then the study of language use, of the structure and characteristics of discourse in general and specific discourse genres in particular. The term 'text linguistics', is used by some (van Dijk, 1972, de Beaugrande and Dressler, 1981) to refer to the study of language use, both spoken and written.

Since the influences which shape instances of language in use (discourse) are numerous, the study of these influences and the structures they create (discourse analysis), is essentially multidisciplinary in nature. In his introduction to the first volume of his Handbook of Discourse Analysis (volumes 1–4), van Dijk (1985a–d) refers to discourse analysis as 'a new cross-discipline'. Discourse analysis is perceived as an all-embracing term to capture the shared interest of a wide variety of disciplines for language use, for structure of both written and spoken texts or discourse, for conversational interaction and such. Discourse analysis is studied by such apparently diverse disciplines as anthropology, linguistics, philosophy, psychology, sociology, cognitive science, semiotics, poetics and mass communication research, which share an interest in human communication. Consequently, discourse analysis covers a diversity of topics: conversational turn-taking; intonation in discourse; argumentation; narration and story telling; cognitive strategies in processing of discourse; analysis of protocols; political and ideological discourse; interpersonal conflict; gender; power; cross-cultural communication; non-verbal communication.

Despite such a variety of angles and interests in the study of discourse, common analytical goals and features exist. Two main dimensions of discourse analysis can be identified (van Dijk, 1985e). One focuses on the structural aspects of discourse. Discourse genres are studied in terms of superstructures ('super-syntax'), as a product or a verbal object. Thus, structural characteristics such as initiation-response, opening-middle-closing sequences and cohesive chains (Chapter 3) are identified and described. This structural approach to discourse developed in the 1970s as a reaction to sentence grammars to examine linguistic structure above the sentence (Sinclair and Coulthard, 1975). Sentences and utterances are not linked to form discourse in a haphazard and non-systematic way but have structure and order, comparable to that within sentences.

Since 'utterances are not just static verbal objects but ongoing dynamic accomplishments, that is, forms of action' (van Dijk, 1985f, 3), discourse analysis has also a functional dimension to it. Discourse evolves and unfolds within social structures and cognitive constraints and these processes can also be considered as the domain of discourse analysis. Within its widest interpretation, discourse analysis does not only consider the medium of language but also all other modes (e.g. non-verbal, paralinguistic, proximics) of communication.

Defined as such, it is clear that the term discourse analysis is a very wide-ranging term. It seems to embrace many fields of inquiry such as sociolinguistics, psycholinguistics, ethnomethodology, cognitive psychology, to name but few. In doing so, it constitutes the overriding study of human communication beyond 'linguistics proper', focusing on larger structures and the processes by which they come into being. This perception of discourse analysis is by no means the only one. There is a school of 'linguistically based' discourse analysis (e.g. Sinclair and Coulthard, 1975, Brown and Yule, 1983, Stubbs, 1983, Hoey, 1983) which focuses primarily on the structural analysis of connected spoken and written discourse. This is not however to imply that such approaches concentrate solely on structure. In the description of discourse structure, one inevitably needs to make some reference to how the structures evolve in the dynamics of communication. For instance, when analysing initiation-response structures one needs to consider whether an utterance was intended and interpreted as an initiation or a response.

The structural approach to discourse analysis can be considered a 'level of analysis' similar to levels of linguistic analysis. It can be viewed as a level of analysis above syntax in the linguistic analytical hierarchy. If we consider linguistic hierarchy as being based on the idea of composition, in the same way as phonemes are components of morphemes, which are components of words, which are components of sentences, then the components of discourse structure are sentences and utterances. In the same way that sentences have their structure-dependent conditions of well-formedness, discourse structures have their context-dependent and genre-specific conditions of well-formedness and appropriateness. It needs to be emphasized that the study of 'pragmatics' is not a level of analysis in the sense described here (cf. McTear and Conti-Ramsden, 1989). Rather, pragmatics constitutes a study which draws upon the various levels of linguistics for its data; a study which explores how the various levels of language are used for communicative ends.

How does all of this relate to the study of pragmatics, which can also be defined as an all-embracing study of human communication? The functional approach to discourse and the study of pragmatics have the same interest in how communication evolves and unfolds in human interaction. Pragmatics can be considered more narrowly to focus on the intention (speech acts, Chapter 3) behind utterances, on how this intention is interpreted and on what effect it has on the encounter (e.g. Ferrara, 1985) and as such pragmatics can be considered as an aspect of the functional approach to discourse analysis. It is not our purpose here to enter a detailed discussion of how various disciplines relate to one another, but to draw attention to the fact that the same terms can be used to describe slightly different aspects of the communicative phenomenon or different terms the same phenomenon. We will be using the term 'discourse' to refer to any instances of communication (e.g. piece of discourse = piece of communication), the term 'discourse structure' to refer to the structure of verbal and non-verbal meaning expressions which link to form larger chunks of discourse and the term 'discourse analysis' to refer to the description of discourse structure. As such, discourse analysis concentrates on the product rather than the processes by which the product comes into being. As pointed out above, this does not imply that structural descriptions need not make reference to contextual and procedural influences bearing upon meaning creation. We shall then use the term 'pragmatics' as the all-encompassing term for how all aspects of communication come into existence.

Why make a distinction between structural and functional aspects of discourse? The manipulation of structure and function are likely to have foundations in different human abilities and as such have potentially different implications for the clinical management of communication disorders. In order to be able to handle discourse structure one needs to understand that there are units which need to be, and can be, combined in certain ways in order to be well-formed. One needs to appreciate that structures are motivated and rule-governed. In reference to discourse structure, one needs to know the basic means of linking meanings together into coherent wholes and also the specific structural features of discourse genres. Knowing the rules or principles which generate discourse structures one can produce novel instances of genre-appropriate discourse. For instance, knowing the structural characteristics of the discourse genres of a list, a letter of complaint or an invitation enables one to produce novel instances of these genres when required. Being able to produce communicative lists, letters and invitations involves functional or pragmatic considerations such as what one is aiming to achieve, who the audience is, what can be processed by the recipients, how much needs to be explicitly said and what can be presupposed besides discourse structural knowledge. Such functional ability is founded in one's ability to combine various types of knowledge in order to implement a plan to achieve personal and communicative goals (further pragmatic knowledge, Chapter 5).

CLINICAL PRAGMATICS

The study of human communication, in all its forms and facets, is of prime importance to the speech-language clinician. If we consider the field of pragmatics in its widest of interpretations, it provides practising clinicians and researchers with an all-encompassing framework for studying communicative ability and inability as dynamically developing and functioning entities. What we call 'Clinical Pragmatics' explores:

1. How methods and principles from the fields of pragmatics and discourse analysis can be applied in clinical management of communication disorders;
2. A framework focusing on the influences which bear upon communicative behaviour in the context of communication disorders; a framework which enables one to piece together components of communication in order to explore communication as a whole.

The intentions underlying meaning expressions and the effect of expressions on listeners and communicative contexts have clinical consequences and implications. Similarly, the ideas of effectiveness, style, negotiation of meanings and sharing of responsibility in communication are concepts with clinical relevance. These issues will be addressed in this volume. In addition, the domain of discourse structure and its applicability in the clinical context are considered within a clinical pragmatic approach. The motivations for the inclusion of this are more practical than theoretical. The domain of 'Clinical Discourse Analysis' is considered here because it is an area of communication which tends to be included in 'clinical pragmatic protocols' (e.g. Prutting and Kirchner, 1983). This reflects the interdependence of pragmatics and discourse analysis and their shared interest in meaning in context (i.e. discourse). It also distinguishes discourse analysis and pragmatics from the study of linguistics which considers language structure in largely decontextualized terms. However, in line with recent developments in the clinically oriented sub-disciplines such as Clinical Linguistics (Crystal, 1981) or Clinical Phonology (Grunwell, 1987), Clinical Discourse Analysis constitutes a study in its own right. Yet, attempts at separating two such closely related fields of study could be an impossible enterprise. Thus, subsuming discourse analysis within the domain of Clinical Pragmatics does not enable us to explore it in the detail that it deserves.

Within the study of clinical pragmatics, we shall also acknowledge the need for a framework which enables one to explore how communicative success and failure come into being as a result of an interaction of a variety of factors. When studying communication, be it in normal or clinical populations, we are essentially concerned with the process by which communication comes into being. When studying this process we are concerned with what the speaker and the listener need to know and need to be able to do for communication to be successful, and conversely what the speaker/listener did not know and/or was not able to do for communication to be unsuccessful (pragmatic knowledge and pragmatic competence, Chapter 5). Study of communication problems within a process framework of communication constitutes the study of **clinical pragmatics**. Its goal is to characterize clients' communicative behaviour and ability with a view to diagnosis and remediation by considering not only the role of the client in communication but also of the context of situation and of those interacting with the client. As will be strongly emphasized throughout this book, the view of communicative ability and disability, and success and failure, can become obscured if we concentrate on the client alone and place the heaviest communicative responsibility on the client's shoulders.

RELEVANCE TO SPEECH PATHOLOGY AND THERAPY

Historical perspective

In order to understand the effect of the 'pragmatics revolution' upon clinical practice it is necessary to be aware of the developmental history of the profession concerned.

Organized attempts to help people who have difficulty in communicating have their origins in the present century. The observation of communicative disability in soldiers returning from active service and in civilians subjected to the modern extension of combat areas is widely held to have provided the motivation for studies of language pathology in several countries. These studies were at first conducted by practising physicians and medical scientists. These were followed by individuals such as Charles Van Riper (1939) in the US and Muriel Morley (1957) in the UK who, with others, pioneered the exploration of communicative disability in the absence of a great deal of linguistic or psychological theory, but with generous measures of human understanding, observation and medical information. Logopedists and speech therapists, correctionists or pathologists began to be employed from about the middle of this century with varying degrees of recognition, success and accountability.

Teachers of the deaf and aphasiologists have always, by necessity, concerned themselves with syntax, vocabulary and a wide range of linguistic skills. Remedial speech teachers and clinicians, on the other hand, concerned themselves at one time more with their clients' voice, pronunciation or fluency and communication. The aim of treatment was to enable individuals to communicate in a manner that would be comprehensible and socially acceptable in their own social milieu. There was less awareness then of the possibilities of social mobility. Considerable emphasis was placed upon emotional factors and upon gaining rapport with 'patients' in order to secure co-operation, enhance their self-esteem and improve their confidence in communicative situations. Comparatively little attention was given at that stage to syntactic structures and their production. Linguists sometimes ask how it was possible for speech clinicians to achieve results at a time when they 'knew so little about language', to which a reply might be that language is only one of many areas which speech clinicians manage and need to understand (Chapter 1).

With the growth of linguistic science and in response to the influence of Bloomfield (1933) and the work of Laura Lee (1969, 1974) in the US and David Crystal (1972) in the UK, speech clinicians gained confidence in their ability to assess and treat problems in sentence construction. Unfortunately it was not usual at that time to specify whether the term 'language disorder', which was by then widely used, referred to what the listener heard (i.e. disordered language) or to some hypothesized disorder in the patient's linguistic ability. This failure has caused considerable confusion which is still evident in the literature (Leonard, 1987). Under the influence of Dunn (1959) vocabulary (albeit passive, comprehended vocabulary) was assessed, though less often treated. Reynell (1977), in the UK, provided a means of comparing an individual's language comprehension and production skills. The Reynell Developmental Language Scales have been, and still are, very widely used, even though, linguistically, they perhaps raise more questions than therapists have been prepared to answer. Lee (1969) and Crystal, Fletcher and Garman (1976) provided the means of greatly extending clinical awareness of syntactic issues and the profiling of ability. This was later extended (Crystal, 1982) to include the areas of phonology, prosody and semantics.

For some time experienced clinicians had been stressing that remedial work on comprehension and interaction ought to precede that on production of speech and language (Renfrew and Murphy, 1964). Younger clinicians had appeared to accept this, but as more became known about syntax and its acquisition, those whose training had involved the study of linguistics became conscientious about including something which was often called 'work on structures' in clinical programmes, usually emphasizing production. At the same time, understanding of the development of phonology and of phonological disorders was expanding (Ingram, 1976, Grunwell, 1981). Comprehension continued to receive attention, though its complexity was not always appreciated (Bishop, 1987).

In the treatment of dysfluency, voice problems, aphasia and even developmental delay, pressures were felt toward precise, 'scientific', demonstrable and measurable treatment, preferably leading to precise, demonstrable and measurable improvement. Understandably, therefore, a tendency had developed to concentrate remedial attention upon the client's verbal behaviour in the clinical situation and upon his/her perceived speech and language deficits; from these a speech and language curriculum could be derived and the client could be taught more acceptable verbal behaviour. Linguists, notably Crystal, Fletcher and Garman (1976), at this stage were pointing out that clients' abilities were as important, perhaps more important than their short-comings. Clinicians were pleased to be reminded of this and to have support for their efforts to clarify this feature of assessment when talking to parents, physicians and administrators.

Despite this, however, a deficit-centred curricular approach remained firmly in vogue, especially in the field of delayed language development. Children were taught 'their' prepositions, taught 'their' colours, 'moved on' from one type of structure to a more sophisticated one, etc. Schemes and programmes proliferated which mapped out the sort of progress that could be expected and suggested methods by which the child could be persuaded to practise and remember the required linguistic structures. These met with limited success (Leonard, 1981). So language-centred had clinicians' thinking become that even severely aphasic people were usually given language to relearn rather than being helped to communicate; when this proved less than satisfactory, the value of therapy per se was naturally called into question.

Under the influence of Chomsky (1957; 1965), concentration on the syntactic structures of language reached its peak (see formal approach above); at the same time, however, new emphasis was placed upon children themselves as active, if pre-programmed, learners. If the normal child acquired knowledge of language in a series of astonishing leaps, rather than having to proceed slowly one step at a time, perhaps some at least of our clients could be helped to do the same? It began to appear likely that in the case of both children and adults, we could be dealing with some whose 'language acquisition device' (Chomsky 1965, 32) had been tragically damaged to the extent that pre-programming was no longer effective but with others who had failed to leap for quite different reasons; these latter might still do so, given favourable circumstances. Another possibility seemed to be that some of our clients, while not performing adequately, had adequate competence in Chomsky's sense and were awaiting mobilization of existing powers (Chapter 5). Furthermore, this might be true at a variety of linguistic levels and would call for a communication-centred approach to treatment rather than one centred upon a language curriculum.

Now, in the post-Chomskian era, attention has been redirected to focus on the environment within which learners of a language set about detecting its rules, restrictions and regularities, and upon the question of precisely how the

sharing of meaning takes place at any age. Linguists, anthropologists and social psychologists have returned to
questions about the relationship between language, thought
and social organization and about the potential of both
human and artificial intelligence. Clinicians therefore have
the opportunity to incorporate insights from this work into
existing treatment approaches and to make use of new
hypotheses arising out of it for clinical research. Theore-
ticians, on the other hand, have become more likely to
hybridize the various academic disciplines involved in
the study of language and its uses and effects. Finally,
researchers have become aware that both the study of
language acquisition and that of language disability can
provide insights of a general nature and have therefore
offered themselves as partners to remedial professionals.

Speech pathology and the pragmatics revolution

Clinicians on the whole have welcomed the idea of returning to a consideration of communication, interaction, shared
meanings, personal values, extralinguistic behaviour and
regard for the motivation and active involvement of the
client; many had retained their interest in such matters
regardless of fashionable preoccupations with the form
of language, while others experienced a reawakening of
interest in remedial work once a departure from strictly
speech- and language-centred approaches became legit-
imized. Clinicians had long been accused of adopting a
mechanistic approach to communication problems, and it
was with pleasure and relief that the broader perspectives
of psycholinguistics and pragmatics were in turn adopted.
Gallagher and Prutting (1983) provide clear indications of
how clinical thinking was developing. However, there are
good reasons why the professions most closely concerned
with remediation of communicative disability have exercised
some caution in accepting a totally pragmatics-orientated
view.

In the first place, what has proved partially successful
over the years is not easily abandoned. A problem here
is that measures of success in remediation are difficult to

devise, since one can never be certain whether or not an improvement in one area has contributed to improvement in another. This is particularly true of work on pragmatics (Lucas, 1980). This being so, it is difficult to argue that although some improvement took place using method A, a greater improvement would not have been obtained by using method B. This problem urgently requires investigation if clinical work is to be costed and, more importantly, optimized. Another difficulty for clinicians is that the concept of professionalism involves payment for work. It also currently incorporates the notion that the professional is in charge of the interaction, is carrying the responsibility for initiating what takes place and is liable for any failure in interaction. Pragmatic principles, on the other hand, postulate shared responsibility for interactions and suggest that there are certain rules and requirements for satisfactory interchange which involve subtle and courteous role shifting, mutual adjustment and responsiveness (Grice, 1975, 1978, Wardhaugh, 1985).

It may be the case that handing over some of the responsibility for the interaction, responding to the client, allowing silences and refraining from direct instruction will provide much greater benefit to the client's use of language or to his or her communicative skills than more didactic approaches, but for the following reasons clinicians may feel reluctant to experiment. This behaviour neither feels nor appears professional; it is hard to justify to people unfamiliar with the pragmatics literature; it may take some time to show results and it is at odds with the conventional view of 'patients' and especially the very young as passive, incompetent and potentially lazy, disruptive or manipulative. A rethinking of the role-relationship toward interactive partnership is demanded, and yet this has not been catered for in professional education or, to any great extent, in the literature. Accountability problems are raised whether one is employed privately, and thus to some extent by insurance companies, or by a public body. Questions of self-esteem and conscience also arise for many clinicians in this connection. An added difficulty is that even for those who would like to establish a more interactive relationship with clients, there is a shortage of models or descriptions clarifying exactly how this is done, what to expect, what the altered nature of professional responsibility will be, etc. Particularly in the case of child therapy it is noticeable that some clinicians are unaware that there is an intermediate path between total permissiveness on the one hand and complete adult domination on the other; this is regrettable since it deprives them of enjoyment in young people's company and deprives the young people of essential feed-back as to the reasonableness, or otherwise, of their natural behaviour. Once it is understood that the majority of children are basically sensible and that a courteous, responsive approach to them need not involve tolerating excessively abrasive behaviour, any more than it would with a friend, we shall be able to experiment in comparative comfort, (Miller, 1983, Letts, 1985, Smith, 1988, 1989). To do so is essential in view of research findings clearly showing that generalization of language skills taught to passive recipients outside the normal communicative context is poor and that children communicate less readily where adults are highly directive; Leonard (1981) and Snow (1984) provide valuable summaries of relevant research. To argue, as directive clinicians tend to do, that the communicatively impaired child cannot be expected to take an initiating role in interaction may be premature. One final objection to holistic, communicative therapy could be that, while mechanistic approaches to human activity may be deplorable in philosophical terms, they may make good sense, at least in the early stages of treatment, when a mechanism is faulty. Research is needed to determine whether, and to what extent, this is the case.

The essential difference made to clinical practice by the arrival of 'pragmatics' is that, whilst all the above reservations about interactive therapy are sensible, they are no longer able to hold sway without being questioned. Clinicians who would like to experiment with new approaches or who are dissatisfied with results in a particular area of their work are now able to call upon a growing volume of literature for support. Diagnosis is another major area in which knowledge of pragmatics has been influential by focusing attention on communicative use of language. It may become necessary to reconsider the need for diagnostic labels in the context of pragmatic disturbance, given the complex nature of pragmatic functioning (Chapter 5).

Inevitably this book concentrates more heavily on certain areas of application than others. This is because of our own professional experience. It is for others to develop those areas that we have neglected.

Chapter 3

Analysing discourse

Having outlined what communication involves and how the fields of pragmatics and discourse analysis examine communicative phenomena, we can now discuss in more detail how communicative events have been studied using the methods and principles of pragmatics and discourse analysis. We shall examine those aspects of language use and discourse structure which have been discussed in the literature on communicative handicap in order to provide a background for later chapters on assessment, diagnosis and treatment (Chapters 5, 6 and 7).

SPEECH ACTS

Speech act theory, originally formulated by Austin (1962) and Searle (1969), is one of the most studied areas within pragmatics and an area which is extensively applied to the study of child language and communicative handicaps. Since speech act theory forms a part of almost every book on discourse and pragmatics, we shall not discuss its principles here in any detail, but will direct the reader to the original texts and to such introductory books as Levinson (1983), Leech (1983), Coulthard (1985) and Taylor and Cameron (1987). After a brief outline of the basic features of the theory here, we shall focus upon issues which are particularly pertinent to the communication pathology context.

It is part of human relationships to use language not simply to describe the world around one, but also to initiate and terminate encounters and to let others know one's feelings and wishes. Using language to such social and psychological ends constitutes, in Austin's terms, a speech act. Speaking does not simply entail saying something, but doing something by saying. Thus, saying 'I haven't played for a long time' may function as a statement of fact or it may constitute an act of apology for a bad round of golf ('I'm sorry for giving you such a lousy game'). In this way, a distinction between statements and performatives can be made, the latter implying the performance of some speech act beyond simply describing. While originally Austin did not consider statements as speech acts, he later maintained that statements were speech acts like any others. There is however a dimension which distinguishes statements from other acts. Statements can be true or false while other performatives cannot be judged by these criteria. With regard to the above example then, as a statement we can ascertain whether the person had not played within what is considered a long time in golf, while as an apology it is meaningless to describe it as true or false. An apology can of course be sincere or insincere (or felicitous or unfelicitous; Searle, 1969).

According to Austin, when producing an utterance, a person is performing three 'acts' simultaneously

1. A locutionary act – this refers to the actual production of the words with meaning and reference.
2. An illocutionary act – this refers to the utterance having a particular communicative function or force (illocutionary force) such as apologizing, challenging, informing, warning etc.
3. A perlocutionary act – this refers to the utterance having a particular effect (perlocutionary effect) on the mental state or the behaviour of the listener (e.g. the listener accepting or rejecting an apology).

These acts constitute the total speech act. The locutionary act falls within the domain of linguistics, and in particular of semantics. Pragmatics, being interested in the relationship of meaning to speakers, listeners and contexts, focuses on the illocutionary and perlocutionary acts. Indeed, mutuality of meaning in communication rests upon both illocution and perlocution. While both of these aspects of the total speech act are clearly central to communication, much of the literature has concentrated on the illocutionary act and how it is reflected in language. The perlocutionary act, understandably, has been subjected to less study given the difficulty of examining a phenomenon which is not necessarily explicitly expressed. Illocutionary forces can be recognized in language structures and expressions, in particular in the presence of explicit illocutionary verbs ('I warn you'). There are obviously many utterances in which the intended force is not explicitly expressed and which pose problems for characterizing illocutions in linguistic terms (Levinson, 1983). Perlocutionary effects are even less accessible and more unpredictable. Even an explicit warning can have the effect of not only warning, but also, say, challenging, amusing and annoying, depending on the specific listener and the context.

These points summarize the main import of speech act theory: utterances have meaning beyond the actual words used and their syntactic arrangement and communication occurs at the levels of illocution and perlocution. As such, speech act theory highlights the need to consider utterances not only in terms of their linguistic form but as evolving entities in social interaction, having specific function and being capable of shaping the interaction.

Sentences, as decontextualized entities, do not carry any illocutionary force, but rather illocutionary force is a property of utterances in context. Thus, we cannot determine which speech act is performed without recourse to the appropriate context. 'I haven't played for a long time' can, for instance, function not only as an apology but also as a request for a game, as a refusal of a game, as a request for explanation of rules or as a challenge to play well, depending on the intention behind the utterance in the particular context. Using this utterance to perform any of the above speech acts is a very indirect way of communicating one's intentions. Alternatively, one could have chosen to say 'I'm sorry I gave you such a lousy game', 'Would you like a round of golf?', 'I really don't feel like playing today', 'I haven't played for a long time but I won't let it affect my game' or 'I have forgotten the rules, so would you explain them to me'. Choosing a direct or an indirect speech act depends on a variety of factors. Being direct, while potentially maximally effective in terms of exchange of information, may convey other meanings. One may be perceived as impolite, abrupt, or tactless. Or, on the other hand, direct expression may be equated with honesty, reliability and trustworthiness. Using indirect speech acts can function as a face saving device by offering an easier possibility of later denial ('I never actually promised to do it'). Directness of expression varies in relation to socio-cultural contexts and participant relationships. Being able to choose a direct or an indirect mode of expression appropriately is part of one's pragmatic competence (Chapters 1 and 5).

According to what has been said thus far, every utterance can be classified in terms of its illocutionary force (speech act). There are two further points concerning categorization of utterances which need be made. Firstly, given that there is an indefinite number of different contexts in which utterances can occur and given that illocutionary force is context dependent, then there cannot be a predetermined set of speech acts. Yet, cultures and sub-cultures share many of the same contexts and thus similar speech acts are likely to occur. What, however, needs to be emphasized is that different individuals may attribute different illocutionary force to the same utterance, even in the same context because of the nature of their frame of reference. Thus, ultimately there is no right or wrong categorization, although much consensus can be found amongst like-minded individuals. One must not forget, however, that one can choose to mis-interpret the illocutionary force of utterances for one's own purposes.

Most writers consider each utterance as carrying one illocutionary force (i.e. categorized in terms of one speech act). Yet, we commonly talk about deeper meanings or hidden messages carried by utterances. In their investigations of therapeutic discourse, Labov and Fanshel (1977) came to the conclusion that most utterances perform several speech acts at any one time. They proposed that such speech act hierarchies can be analysed in terms of a level of superficiality or abstractness. It is characteristic of therapeutic encounters that therapists listen to underlying meanings, interpreting apparent surface statements as refusals,

challenges, denials or such. While the idea of speech act
hierarchies is challenged in the literature (e.g. Edmondson,
1981, Taylor and Cameron, 1987), it appeals to one's intuitive knowledge of what happens in conversation, and, in
our opinion, is a valuable notion for those dealing with
communicative handicaps. Assume that near examination
time, a lecturer in the course of explaining a point says
'This is a very important point.' Beyond simply stating that
indeed this is a crucial aspect of the topic in question it can
also be interpreted as a request for further reading, a suggestion for revision or even a hint of a possible examination
question. It may not be that every individual would attribute the same illocutionary forces to this utterance but it
is likely that the utterance would carry more than one illocutionary force for some listeners or not the same meanings
for all. Or, consider a clinical situation where a client's
utterance 'My dad has to get angry coz I'm so naughty'
carries the function of request for help ('Please help me.
My dad keeps hitting me'). Failing to appreciate the less
obvious interpretation can have far-reaching implications.

One central aspect of Austin's theory is a link between
speech acts and social roles. For certain speech acts to have
any chance of having the intended perlocutionary effect
they have to be performed by particular individuals. Any
person can utter the words 'I pronounce you man and wife'
but only when uttered by a person authorized to marry
people is this speech act successful (or felicitous, Austin,
1962). Beyond having some fun, no 'normally functioning'
unauthorized person believes they can perform the act of
marrying, christening, naming ships etc. by simply uttering
the words. Apart from such highly conventionalized speech
acts, in theory any person can promise, challenge, refuse,
request, question and perform a variety of other speech
acts. In real human relationships and communicative situations, however, social roles constrain the performance of
speech acts. As one's social roles are defined in relation to
one's current interactive partner, the range of speech acts
which can be performed is likely to differ for any individual
in different communicative situations. This observation is of
crucial importance for those working with the communicatively handicapped. It would not be a surprise, for instance,

if a child did not request information, did not challenge or perform other such assertive speech acts in encounters with authority figures. Awareness of the nature of the client-therapist relationship and the possible constraints it may place on the client's communicative functioning enables one to work with and around such constraints.

Speech act theory deals almost exclusively with verbal expression of meaning. Yet, utterances often gain illocutionary force as a combination of verbal (including para-linguistic) and non-verbal expressions. Saying 'I am serious' with a steady eye gaze and holding a fist in the air is most likely to be intended and interpreted as a threat. Being able to co-ordinate the different channels of communication to produce the intended communicative force and being able to interpret the intended signal appropriately and to act upon it accordingly requires the variety of abilities described in Chapter 1. Speech acts can also be performed by non-verbal means alone. A simple nod can act as a thank you and that dreaded look by mother with a pointing finger functions as a warning to many children.

Outlined as such, speech act theory provides a suitable means for labelling communicative behaviours within the functional paradigm. It has been used as a descriptive device in a variety of domains of enquiry into communication, including the speech pathology context. In assessment of pragmatic functioning (Chapter 6), the methodology commonly involves labelling of utterances as questions, answers, statements, challenges, requests etc. Studying communication within this framework highlights how utterances are used in social contexts. It can reveal restricted ranges of communicative functions performed by seemingly verbose clients or conversely the richness of speech acts performed by handicapped individuals with very limited language. However, there are issues which have been largely ignored when using speech act frameworks and which can affect the way speech acts are identified and interpreted. To summarize those discussed above

1. Social roles of the participants defined by culture and sub-culture and the over-all communicative context affect the speech acts performed;

2. No predetermined set of speech acts is adequate to describe all communicative contexts;
3. Listeners identify illocutionary force on the basis of their individual frame of reference;
4. Each utterance can perform more than one speech act at any one time, ranging within a scale of explicitness;
5. Speech acts can be performed not only by verbal means but by a combination of verbal, paralinguistic and non-verbal means or by non-verbal means only.

In addition to these points, it is worth noting two further issues concerning speech acts. Firstly, speech acts can materialize as a consequence of a negotiation process (Stubbs, 1983). This is particularly important to note in unequal encounters where the negotiation may be controlled by the partner with the higher status. In the following example the adult can be seen attributing a function to the child's utterance which may not necessarily be there.

C. I might do that tomorrow.
A. Promise?
C. Yeah.
A. Sure?
C. Yeah.

When analysing data in terms of speech act categories it is not clear what to do about instances where the illocutionary force is negotiated. Does the child's original utterance function as a promise? While we cannot answer this, we need to recognize, in particular in clinical contexts, how speech acts come into being and in doing so consider not only the client's contributions but also the dynamics of the whole communication process (Chapters 1 and 6).

Another point relevant to using speech acts as an analytical framework concerns opting out from performing speech acts. Bonikowska (1988) argues for the recognition of the speaker's decision not to perform a speech act as an equally legitimate pragmatic strategy to that of choosing to perform one. In the clinical context, it is necessary to recognize that clients have the right to opt out. The question is, however, whether the absence of speech acts is a reflection of an appropriate opting out strategy, of an inappropriate strategy reflecting problems with pragmatic competence (Chapters 2 and 5), of lack of an opting out strategy (pragmatic knowledge, Chapters 2 and 5) or of contextual constraints which do not allow the client to perform many speech acts. Attempting to provide answers to any of these questions is difficult, yet awareness of the possibility and legimaticy of opting out guards against too readily interpreting lack of behaviours as indicative of lack of ability or the presence of a disorder (Leinonen and Smith, 1989, and Chapter 5).

EXCHANGE STRUCTURE

Utterances can be analysed at different levels of abstraction. Speech acts, as outlined above, examine what the social and psychological functions of utterances may be while the speaker participates in social interaction (makes promises; thanks; greets; teases etc.). The same utterances can be analysed in terms of their function in organizing the discourse itself. Whatever the social function of utterances, they also have a place in a sequence of utterances in discourse. Interactions themselves are organized by initiating, responding and terminating interactional sequences. Such discourse structure is commonly referred to as exchange structure (Sinclair and Coulthard, 1975, discourse acts, Stubbs, 1983). As above, we shall not discuss the exchange structure of discourse in any great detail here, but shall refer the reader to Sinclair and Coulthard (1975), Coulthard and Brazil (1981) and Stubbs (1983) for a more rigorous examination of the topic. Rather, we shall concentrate on the basics and focus on the structure of discourse in clinical encounters.

Pieces of discourse differ from formal sentences by being dynamic entities evolving in communicative contexts, and thus partly acquiring structure from these contexts. Written discourse has a different structure from spoken, as do monologues, dialogues and multiparty conversations. Social roles, communicative situations, the capabilities of the participants and such are likely to affect the structure of discourse. Apart from the differences, much of human discourse is also based on shared needs, conventions and beliefs. Much of this shared experience may be culture or sub-culture bound rather than common to the whole of human kind. The fundamental similarities of human existence can, however, be seen as imposing structural universals in discourse. What exactly these universals might be remains to be studied, yet the basic exchange structure in conversational interaction as studied by Sinclair and others can be viewed as reflecting a possible universal feature.

An exchange is considered the basic structural unit in conversational discourse. A basic exchange structure consists of two elements: initiation and response. This structure reflects the very core of human interaction which is based on somebody doing/saying something and somebody else responding to this action. Initiations and responses can take almost any form: a letter in a newspaper column, a look across a room, a smile, a greeting, an off-chance comment, an explicit question etc. As such, discourse is viewed as consisting of sequences of initiations and responses.

It needs to be noted that the term 'response' can have different interpretations. In most general terms, any act of responding to a stimulus is a response. This is the meaning adhered to in the previous paragraph. However, much of the work done on exchange structure has a narrower frame of interpretation for the term. Sinclair and Coulthard (1975) identified an Initiation-Response-Feedback structure as a basic exchange structure in classroom, teacher-pupil, interaction (see Sinclair and Coulthard for the full analytical framework which is much more complex and comprehensive than implied here).

> T. Can you tell me what this means?   (Initiation)
> P. It means 'you can't drive that way'.   (Response)
> T. That's right.   (Feedback)

In this taxonomy, response signifies the provision of information to a question. Within the broader framework, feedback is also a type of response. We find it more useful to use the term response in the more general terms and then classify responses (and initiations) further to reflect their more refined characteristics. In this way, initiation and response structures are viewed at a higher level of hierarchical description than categories such as question, answer and feedback. At this higher level of abstraction, we can also envisage utterances which function as initiations and responses simultaneously.

> T. Can you tell me what this means?
> P. Does it mean 'you can't drive that way'? (Response/
> T. Yes. Initiation)

Such dual functions of utterances are important for the progress of conversational interaction, by responses providing impetus for further development of a topic. Every response potentially acts as an initiation by triggering further development of a topic or a topic shift or change. This is true if we consider initiations in a broad sense of 'providing impetus for a further utterance'. Some initiations function more clearly as such (e.g. direct questions) while others might need a great deal of processing by the listener in order for one to be able to identify how a response can lead to a further comment. Indeed, an ability to provide responses which can also be easily identified as functioning as initiations may be a defining characteristic of an enjoyable and smooth interaction. McTear (1984) stresses the importance of facilitating children's use of these response/initiations.

We can assume that conversational discourse consists of exchange structures and that the basic exchange structure consists of Initiation-Response sequences which in turn can be realized by different forms and have additional social functions. This is not however to imply that a conversation is a simple sequence of I-R-I-R-I. As is apparent from the first example above, a response can be responded to by providing feedback (I-R-R(F)). Furthermore, reflecting negotiation in discourse, an original initiation may not be responded to until later in the sequence (insertion sequence, Schegloff, 1972, side sequence, Jefferson, 1972).

> A. Isn't this all a bit ridiculous? (I,1)
> B. Why ridiculous? (I,2)
> A. Well, making fools of ourselves. (R,2)
> B. I suppose so. (R,1)

Clarification and repair sequences can provide similar embedded initiation and response structure. Furthermore, not actually saying anything or not otherwise overtly responding can also act as a response.

If a conversation is a sequence of I-R structures, how do we then determine where one exchange ends and another begins? Stubbs (1983) outlines two main criteria for defining conversational exchanges. The first, semantically based definition, defines an exchange as a whole propositional (meaning) unit which completes or closes the information introduced in the initial initiation (also, Coulthard and Brazil, 1981). The second definition, a syntactically based consequence of the first, outlines an exchange in terms of elliptical structures interpretable within the exchange (see cohesion and coherence below). Defined as such, it is clear that conversations are not necessarily sequences of well-defined exchange structures. Initiations are not always responded to nor are topics always brought to a close. This is a point worth noting in clinical interactions in order not to penalize clients who become interested in other topics without bringing previously initiated topics to an end. A difference is likely to be detected between 'normal conversational drifting' and one induced by inadequate pragmatic functioning.

A further point which is central to the notion of conversational exchange, is that initiations may constrain the subsequent responses. A question usually begs an answer, a greeting a counter-greeting, a clarification requests a clarification and so on (adjacency pairs, see Coulthard, 1985). The idea that stimuli may influence the nature of the response is an important one for clinicians. It has been widely recognized that yes-no questions and other closed questions such as 'When is your birthday?' tend to produce minimal answers with little elaboration, while open-ended questions and initiations are more likely to lead to longer turns ('Tell me about . . .'). The conceptual complexity and interest of initiations are also likely to influence the nature of the resultant responses (Brown, 1989). Appreciation of the potential effects of stimuli on responses guards against potential misperception of inappropriate responses or absent responses as indices of pragmatic failure on the part of the client.

OPENING–MIDDLE–CLOSING SEQUENCES

It was observed above that the notion of initiation and response constitutes a possible discourse universal for the genre of conversational interaction. Similarly, many conversations and written texts have the structure of 'opening–middle–closing' or 'beginning–middle–end'. In conversation, this structure is founded in the need to first ascertain that the communication channel is open before making the contributions one wishes to make.

A. 'Hi. All right?'
B. 'Yeah. And you?'
A. 'Yes thanks. Listen, I wanted to ask you . . .'

and many other such utterances and sequences serve the function of opening conversations. Such initial opening statements can be followed by metastatements which specify the nature of the interaction ('I wanted to ask you . . .'; 'I hope you don't think I am too forward but . . .') (see metacommunication, below). Similarly, interactions tend to be closed by some statement rather than simply walking away, putting the phone down or turning one's back. Utterances and sequences such as 'Well, that's about all then', 'Bye. See you soon.'

A. Nice to have talked to you.
B. Yeah. You too.
A. Take care then.
B. You too.
A. Bye bye then.
B. Bye

reflect social convention rather than having other communicative function. Yet, social rules are very powerful regulators of interaction, outcasting those who do not adhere to the principles dictated by convention.

While opening and closing sequences bear important functions in communication, it is in between these where much of meaning is conveyed and where relationships are developed or abandoned. We may not always wish to enter this meaningful middle sequence in discourse; many relationships are based on what can be considered as opening and closing sequences only (e.g. talking to strangers at bus stops; to neighbours). When interacting with the communicatively handicapped discourse may also be based on opening and closing routines. This may simply reflect difficulty of knowing what to say. One may however begin to worry when much of interaction becomes in this way stereotyped and one may need to re-evaluate one's own perception of what interaction involves with the communicatively handicapped.

METACOMMUNICATION

Part of one's communicative ability is to be able to communicate about communication itself. This is referred to as metacommunication (Stubbs, 1983) or metapragmatics (Smith, 1988). Much of communication involves explicit organization of the path the interaction is to take by use of metacommunicative statements. Such statements may serve many functions: they may forewarn the listener about a potential perlocutionary effect ('You will not like what I have to say'); they may serve to change topics ('Could we talk about something more cheerful please?'); they may indicate understanding ('I see what you mean') or lack of understanding ('I'm sorry, I don't understand'); they may repair overlap ('Carry on'); they may serve to control the interaction ('Don't interrupt') and so on. Metacommunicative statements have the overriding function of explicitly organizing the running of conversation. By metacommunication the speaker makes his/her communicative intentions explicit within the confines of social conventions. One cannot produce such metastatements as 'You listen for a change', 'You do talk a lot of rubbish' or even 'What do you mean?' (Stubbs 1983, 58) without the backing of a familiar or authorititive relationship or without appearing inappropriate and rude. It is metacommunication which makes communication run smoothly and thus, conversely, without such 'signposting and policing' communication can be very cumbersome and uncomfortable.

While over-all metacommunication is about being able to monitor the interaction and to act accordingly, we can distinguish between two levels of metacommunicative ability or awareness. Firstly, there is the wide-ranging awareness of what makes communication work or not work, which can, however, involve some very specific knowledge of causes of success and failure. It may involve awareness of topics which upset people ('Whatever you do don't talk about X'), of over-all evaluation of another person's communicative style ('Can't get a word in edge-ways with him') or of projected outcome of the interaction ('I must get him to agree'). This kind of awareness is aware-ness of the defining characteristics of an act of communi-cation in general and in specific situations (Chapter 5). In a way, it forms the background within which specific communicative behaviours manifest themselves and by which they can be improved. Secondly, we can envisage metacommunicative awareness which manifests (or fails to manifest) itself in the heat of the interaction. This could be referred to as metapragmatic awareness. It involves awareness of when to speak or listen ('If you let me finish'; 'Can you add anything?'), of when it is appropriate to inter-rupt ('Now, that's enough'; 'I'm sorry to interrupt but I have to go now'), of the appropriate speech acts ('I'm sorry, I think I've gone too far'; 'I would like to ask at this point . . .') and so on. For successful communication, one needs both metacommunicative and metapragmatic aware-ness and a range of metacommunicative statements to perform the specific metafunctions.

Metacommunication is also an integral part of one's in-ternal discourse. Communication is planned, judged and managed not only overtly but in one's own mind which then guides how the interaction is likely to progress. Such internal metacommunication creates overt communication: it constitutes the planning of the overt interaction. Often such planning is best done in one's mind in order to aid smooth running of discourse and to avoid conflict.

Metacommunication is tied closely to social roles. Part of one's pragmatic competence (Chapters 2 and 5) is the ability to judge who has the right to make metacommunicative statements and when it is appropriate to do so. Conver-sational rights reflect specific participant relationships. They may reflect status differences where one of higher status has the right to monitor the progress of the interaction. By their professional obligations, teachers, clinicians and instructors of any kind feel they ought to control and manage communicative encounters. It is yet another matter whether this right is exercised sensibly or abused and whether this right is conducive to learning of whatever skills one is attempting to teach (Chapter 7). In more equal encounters, metacommunicative rights may be shared or negotiatied. Exploring metacommunication in interaction provides a means of evaluating the nature of the participant relationships and their potential effect on how the interaction develops (Chapters 1 and 4).

One further point made by Stubbs (1983) is of central importance for the clinical context. According to him

> Explicit metacomments on anyone's speech are heard as evaluative in any social context (unless they are heard as doing the legitimate, practical work of checking on understanding or on whether the audience can hear clearly, etc.) (p. 59).

While this observation provides much to think about for the practising clinician, let us first consider what is meant by 'explicit' here. 'Explicit' cannot mean 'direct' as opposed to 'indirect' in that indirect expressions such as 'My hearing's not very good' can function as metacomments (i.e. 'I cannot hear you'). Also, hearing a metacomment such as 'I cannot understand you' as a non-evaluative statement, which it may be intended to be, is dependent on the listener. It is not difficult to imagine a foreign language learner or a communicatively handicapped person interpreting such a comment as evaluative in relation to their powers of expression.

If metacomments which are not genuine attempts at keeping the channel open are perceived as evaluative, the question is whether the numerous metacommunications of clinicians are intended as such and have this function for the client. One of the basic principles of therapy is not to judge and evaluate too harshly and unnecessarily, and thus potentially diminish the client's confidence, but to provide a supportive and encouraging learning context (see Chapter 7). Could it then be that clinicians evaluate by their metacommunicative behaviour without being totally aware of doing so? By taking full responsibility for the management of the communicative interaction by such metacommunicative behaviours as turn allocation and requests for repetition and by non-adherence to many of the 'normal' communicative principles (Clinical Interaction, below), do clinicians evaluate the client as a non-capable communicator? Examining issues such as these and balancing the outcomes with the clinicians' task of facilitating learning of new behaviours is a step towards a realistic appraisal of the strengths and weaknesses of the clinical encounter.

DISCOURSE ANALYSIS OF CLINICAL INTERACTION

Having discussed some means of looking at discourse phenomena, it is useful at this point to examine how these ideas have been applied in the analysis of clinical interactions. We would like to consider briefly the nature of conversational exchanges in tightly structured (Chapter 7) speech therapy sessions. This exploration is based mainly on McTear (1985a), Letts (1985), Panagos, Bobkoff and Scott (1986) and Panagos, Bobkoff-Katz, Kovarsky and Prelock (1988).

The clinical 'lesson' has many parallels with the lesson in the classroom in terms of who controls the exchange, the types of initiations and responses performed by the participants and the goals and likely outcomes. The clinical interaction is often motivated by the aim to aid learning of linguistic structures. Tightly structured therapy does not often attempt to facilitate communicative skills beyond linguistic learning (Chapter 7). The therapist tends to operate with preplanned activities which focus on particular aspects of speech and language. Other factors which influence the interactional style include the physical context of the therapy room and the social roles of the participants. Therapy rooms are often small with tables, chairs and materials such as toys and pictures. Most commonly, the therapist and the client sit at a table focusing on specific pictures and objects on the table. The social roles of the therapist and the client are fixed, assigning to the therapist the power to control and manage the interaction (e.g. turn taking and topic) and the client the obligation to co-operate and respond. Interestingly, the therapist need not co-operate with the client having the right to ignore or interrupt the client's contributions (cf. Grice's co-operative principle, Chapter 1). Therapists also tend to adhere closely to a clinical speech register which is characterized by a firmer and louder voice, simpler sentence structure, slower and more precise delivery and minimal smiling and laughter. Clinical interactions have been compared, in our view rather descriptively, to an interview (Bishop and Adams, 1989).

Within this background, discourse structure and pattern in the clinical session emerge. This structure has been described in terms of hierarchically structured units (Letts, 1985, Panagos *et al.* 1986, 1988). Within a session, opening, 'work' and closing phases can be identified. The initial opening phase, of short duration, consists of greetings, small talk, taking off coats, arranging seating and other pre-task activities. The 'work' phase involves the actual therapy and thus lasts the longest and involves pre-planned activities. The closing phase, like the opening phase, is short, consisting of summaries, reminders, putting on coats and goodbyes.

The actual clinical teaching phase has been analysed in terms of the exchange structure and types of speech (communicative) acts. The basic exchange structure is the same initiation-response-feedback pattern as identified in teacher-pupil interaction by Sinclair and Coulthard (1975). Within this structure, the therapist mainly initiates and gives feedback and it is the role of the client to respond to the initiations. As Letts (1985) points out, a child client in particular is in the rather passive role of respondent whose spontaneous contributions, seen as incompatible with the on-going activity, tend not to be elaborated upon. Research has primarily examined the verbal behaviour of therapists in more detail and thus we shall now briefly consider the kinds of speech acts commonly realizing the therapist's initiation and feedback exchanges. Considering these in more detail highlights the therapist-oriented nature of clinical interactions in a more obvious way.

Letts (1985) divides the speech (communicative) acts used by therapists into organizing acts and on-going acts. The former have the function of initiating activity and ensuring its smooth running. The latter acts, on the other hand, serve the purposes of eliciting specific responses, giving feedback on them and giving more general information. The organizing and on-going acts can be analysed further to reflect more specific behaviours (Letts, 1985).

Organizing
1. initiate activity
   - Boundary markers: indicate that a new activity is to happen (e.g. 'Right'; 'Now' with a falling intonation).
   - Orientations: explain what the activity involves ('You tell me about these pictures').
2. ensure the smooth running of the activity.
   - Attention getters: gain/regain attention before initiation ('Listen carefully'; 'Christopher'; 'Watch').
   - Behaviour modifiers: inhibit unwanted behaviours ('Sit still'; 'Come back here'; 'Take your thumb out').
   - Comprehension checks: check that initiation is understood ('OK' with a rising intonation; 'Do you see?'; 'Got it?')
   - Requests for repetition: ('Pardon?'; 'Can you say that again?')

Ongoing
1. elicit specific responses
   - Directives: elicit mainly non-verbal responses ('Point to the picture with a girl in it'; 'Can you stick your tongue out like this'; 'Say "spin"').
   - Questions: seek information unknown or known (testing) to the therapist ('What do you usually do on Saturdays?'; 'What colour is a sunflower?').
   - Signals: involve requests for imitation, signals as prompts requiring a response ('Spin' requiring imitation; 'The man is . . .' requiring completion; pointing at a picture requiring naming).
2. Feedback: usually more positive than negative ('That's right'; 'Good boy').
3. Give general information ('It's like a balloon but much bigger.')

While Letts emphasizes the verbal means of conveying the particular functions, she also recognizes the role of non-verbal behaviour in clinical interactions. Gestures, facial expressions, paralinguistic features, posture and the like signal meanings which are communicative to the client. Panagos *et al.* (1988) provide a detailed study of non-verbal behaviour in clinical encounters. One aspect which is worth emphasizing here is the role of non-verbal signals in communicating one's feelings and attitudes. A crucial aspect of therapy is a 'real' relationship between the therapist and the client and non-verbal behaviours constitute a subtle means of establishing such a relationship. Physical proximity, touch or smiling might be seen as helpful, while sheltering behind a desk or keeping one's eyes on the record sheet can act as powerful signals to the client that he/she is only another case which the therapist is working on.

As is apparent, this analytical framework incorporates concepts from speech act theory, the notion of exchange structure and the idea of larger discourse frames. Focusing solely on the therapist is obviously only part of the picture. For one to be able to determine whether therapy based on such structured discourse works, whether it aids linguistic learning and whether it addresses problems in more general communicative handicaps, an interactive framework of analysis is needed. Examining what effect the therapist's communicative behaviours have on the client, how the client responds to the different stimuli and how the client's communicative behaviours come into being as a reflection of the clinical interaction is a step toward a more realistic appraisal of the clinical encounter. Smith (1989) and Chapters 7 and 8 in the present volume provide an alternative model of therapeutic interaction.

TURN TAKING

One aspect of conversational interaction is that the participants take turns at speaking and listening. Turn-taking dynamics of conversations were first described by the sociologists Sacks, Schegloff and Jefferson (1974), whose ideas have been applied to the study of many types of interactions, including those of communicatively handicapped populations (Chapters 5 and 6). Description of the mechanics of turn changes, possible overlaps, silences and interruptions provides another analytical framework for studying discourse. Some basic characteristics of turn taking were described in Chapter 1 under the sub-heading of 'Reciprocity in Communication'. We shall now expand on this discussion. The reader is also directed to Coulthard (1985) for a succinct summary of conversational turn taking.

When studying turn taking we are essentially interested in:

1. How the speaker indicates to the listener that he/she wants to yield the floor;
2. How the change of role of speaker/listener proceeds;
3. How silences are dealt with;
4. How overlap is dealt with;
5. How interruptions are dealt with.

Turn taking is based on the premise that turns are valued in conversation and that at least one person but not more than one person speaks at any one time. It is thus clear that turn taking is a complex co-operative process in which the speaker and the listener try to co-ordinate their contributions so that overlap and silences are minimized, or feel comfortable for the interactants. Speakers and listeners have means of remediating situations where turns overlap or extended silences occur. Let us consider (1) to (5) briefly and consider their implications for the clinical context.

Theoretically, a speaker's turn is never complete as far as the listener is concerned. The speaker can always add more to their turn, even if an end of turn has been signalled. In practice, however, this is not the case. At one level, the speaker may run out of topics at any given moment and at another, speakers and listeners participate in conversation with the assumption that more than one person makes a contribution and that any one turn is not unreasonably lengthy. Yet, it is true that the listener can never be certain whether the speaker has finished or has more to add. Because of this basic uncertainty, the listener looks for possible points of completion rather than actual points of completion. In doing so the listener looks for particular speaker signals which may indicate that the speaker is coming to an end.

Speaker signals can be fairly subtle or direct (e.g. Duncan,

1972). A complete idea or topic or a grammatically complete sentence can signal to the listener that they could take the floor (but see coherence below). Paralinguistic indices such as falling intonation, drop in pitch or loudness and a drawl on the final syllable can indicate end of a turn too. Similarly, a prolonged pause (maybe only a few seconds) indicates to the listener that the speaker either has run out of things to say or that he/she is planning a further utterance, either case however offering the listener the chance to take the floor. Similar meanings are communicated by repetition of previous information and by explicit offering of the floor by, for instance, asking a question. Also, use of stereotypical utterances such as 'you know' or 'or something like that' can function as end-of-turn signals. The speaker has also non-verbal signals at their disposal. For instance, speakers are observed to have a pattern of short eye contact and looking away in the middle of turns and prolonged eye contact as turns come to an end (Kendon, 1967). Speakers have also been observed to stop hand gesticulation or relax tensed hands or posture at the end of turns (Duncan and Fiske, 1977). Listeners observe these kinds of signals and attempt to determine when it is time for them to take the floor.

In most informal conversations any one person's turn is relatively short, possibly of the duration of only a few utterances. The speaker can, however, attempt to extend their turn by the use of certain discourse devices. Beginning one's turn by 'Let me tell you what happened to me last night' or 'Have you heard the one about . . .' signals to the listener that the speaker is intending to keep the floor for an extended period. Similarly, starting with a subordinate conjunction such as 'if' or 'whenever' claims a turn of at least two clauses. A further method, often employed in political discussions, attempts to guarantee a longer turn by utterances such as 'I'd like to make three points' or simply and more flexibly, 'Firstly'. Interestingly, such expressions often seem to serve the main purpose of reserving some floor space prior to the actual planning of the content of the turn, and thus it is not unusual for the speaker not to adhere to the number of points they had initially declared they intended to make.

A further function of such metacommunicative utterances is to force listeners, who do not respect the reservation for an extended turn, into the role of interrupter which may carry social connotations of being aggressive and self-centred. While some of these adjectives may well describe some listeners, we might also refer to such people in more positive terms such as assertive, confident and ones who know their conversational rights. Similarly, by claiming an extended turn, speakers signal to others their own perception of self-worth and a degree of confidence, with the underlying message of 'I have something to say which I think is worthwhile and which I think you should listen to'. Unfortunately, our own perception of what is worth listening to does not always coincide with that of others: we all know people who monopolize the floor. The reasons for this can vary from one's perception of one's professional obligation (speech therapists?) to lacking the confidence to stop. The latter may seem a curious state of affairs yet it captures the verbosity of some who are perceived as having little of value to contribute. Also, it may reflect why 'normally functioning' individuals tend to monopolize the floor when interacting with the communicatively handicapped: it takes a great deal of confidence to stop and wait for the other's contribution when the wait can be a long one. Conversely, people who rarely make extended turns may signal to others their insecurity and lack of confidence. Or, one may simply prefer brief contributions. Indeed, lack of conversational contributions does not necessarily imply that one does not know how to interact or has no contributions to make but may reflect many other valid reasons (Chapter 5).

Turn taking does not always run smoothly: one turn does not follow another in perfect harmony without silences or overlap. Nor is every turn allowed to be completed without another person claiming the floor by interrupting. Focusing first on silence, it is commonly maintained that silences are not tolerated in discourse. If the listener does not begin shortly after a speaker has fallen silent, remedial strategies tend to be employed (Sacks *et al.*, 1974). The speaker may incorporate the silence into his/her turn by turning the silence into a filled pause ('umm') which then can prompt the listener to take the floor. Or alternatively, the speaker may continue speaking.

While prolonged silences are most probably not tolerated in conversations between relatively unfamiliar individuals or between those who do not feel comfortable with one another, they are an integral part of more comfortable or intimate interactions. Between husbands and wives, between long-term friends, a question may become answered not within a few seconds or so but perhaps within half an hour, if at all. In such relationships there may be no need to ask for permission to be silent while in less familiar relationships one might need to employ some means of incorporating a silence into one's turn ('Let me think about this for a moment'). It is part of one's pragmatic ability to know when and how to seek such permission. Failing to observe this principle can be very destructive for the interaction. One of the current authors converses regularly with a colleague who falls silent quite unexpectedly, often apparently in the middle of a turn. The indecision is whether this person has come to the end of a turn or has just paused to think. At first, the author's strategy was to start speaking which, however, often led to a sharp 'If you let me finish' or even 'If you wouldn't interrupt please'. The latter apparently referring to interrupting one's thinking. This then led to the development of a very direct strategy by the author who now simply asks 'Have you finished?' or 'Are you thinking for the moment?' How one deals with apparent disregard for the basic principles of turn dynamics is dependent on who the violating party is and how well that person is capable of handling apparent criticism. As, in the above instance, it may at times be best for those being disturbed to develop coping strategies rather than jeopardize functioning relationships. Furthermore, those with communicative handicaps may not be able to modify their communication and thus it may have to be those interacting with them who develop adaptation strategies (see also communication strategies below).

The notion of an extended gap between turns is an important one in the clinical context. Owing to the nature of their communicative handicaps, clients may require extra space to process input and to formulate output. It is thus essential for those interacting with handicapped individuals to allow room for processing and as such not to follow the usual turn-taking principles. It is surprisingly difficult to wait for a response in silence. One tends to feel that it is up to one as a 'normally functioning' individual to create the illusion of smooth interaction, which may involve taking the other person's turn or abandoning the need for a contribution.

Taking another person's turn is a likely reflection of the need for 'normal' interaction. It can also reflect one's role as a manager or controller of the conversation. Waiting silently for another person to speak creates such problems as where should one look, should one sit/stand absolutely still, should one indicate to the client non-verbally that one is waiting or try to signal that all is fine, should one nod/smile encouragingly (patronizingly?) and so on. Whatever the answers to these questions might be, those interacting with communicatively handicapped individuals need to learn to cope with such possible uncertainties and feelings of discomfort. There is obviously a point at which one has waited long enough and recognizing these points is based on one's sensitivity and professional experience. While allowing clients adequate space to communicate, one aim of therapy is to reduce this space so that the client can participate in a greater variety of communicative encounters.

The timing of a change of speaker might also cause problems in turn taking. The next speaker can take a turn before the current speaker has stopped speaking or may begin speaking at the same time with another speaker. Overlaps occur at possible points of completion and are, usually, unintentional violations of the other's turn. For communicative effectiveness it is necessary to remedy a situation where two or more people speak simultaneously. There are some general patterns as to how overlaps tend to be remedied (Coulthard, 1985). Assuming that the next speaker overlaps with the current speaker, then the current speaker is likely to finish their turn and the person who caused the overlap is likely to apologize.

A. and I was quite glad ⎱that he came home
B.   ⎰yeah it's . . .
    Sorry

A. Yeah I was glad he decided to come home
B. Umm it's such a relief, isn't it?

Similarly, the current speaker is likely to continue after a pause, during which time another person has begun. A different situation is likely to arise when two people start speaking at the same time after the current speaker has finished a turn. Who carries on depends on factors such as status, power, personality, assertiveness and self-confidence. Those who perceive themselves as lower status or who do not feel confident might simply stop, or apologize and stop, and allow the other person to carry on. People with more equal status and similar personalities may negotiate who carries on ('You carry on'; 'Can I just say this one thing first?') Or the overlapping speakers may compete for the turn, the person who is most persistent, maybe louder and clearer, winning the turn. A situation may also arise where both speakers stop after overlap and start again, and stop and start. Such stop-start sequences may be remedied by a laugh accompanied with a metastatement allocating the next turn.

While overlap in turn taking reflects a timing problem, interruption is an intentional violation of another's turn. As such, interruptions occur in the middle of turns rather than near possible points of completion. An interruption may reflect inappropriate judging of the end of turn. If such interruptions occurred not very near possible points of completion and occurred frequently, a pragmatic problem might be evidenced (Chapter 5). That is to say, that the person has problems of interpreting speaker-signals which indicate the end of turn and/or is not aware of when and how interruption is appropriate. Interruption can be a negative or a positive action depending on whether it is done appropriately or inappropriately. Appropriate interrupting involves some such metacomment as 'I'm sorry to interrupt but . . .'. Knowing when it is necessary to stop one's interlocutor or to direct others' attention to an urgent matter ('The house is on fire!') and how to do it without offending is part of one's pragmatic ability (Chapter 5). Part of this ability is also to know that one can purposely offend by interrupting ('Shut up, will you').

Interruptions are not particularly frequent in everyday non-confrontational conversations and thus such behaviour is not often called for. Who has the right to interrupt is also tied to social roles and situations. It is not uncommon for adults 'to talk over' children, employers over employees, clinicians over clients and younger people over old people. It is less usual for interruptions to occur in the opposite direction in these dyads. It depends on the nature of the participant relationship how the interruption is dealt with. The one being interrupted might simply fall silent, might lessen the impact of the interruption by some such utterances as 'Yes, certainly' or 'Sorry, I didn't realize what the time was' or might react unfavourably ('Now, hang on. Let me finish, if you please'; 'Johnny, for the last time, I warn you'; and/or a non-verbal signal such as direct gaze or frowning).

As is apparent, turn taking is a complex activity which calls upon many skills and abilities (Chapter 1). The turn dynamics described in this section reflect mainly encounters between 'normally functioning' individuals. How is a communicatively handicapped person likely to fare in competing for turns, repairing overlap and asserting their rights by interrupting appropriately? A distinction needs to be drawn between individuals who may not be aware of what they are to do when taking turns or may be aware but cannot judge when and how it is appropriate to do so (Chapter 5). There are also individuals who may be aware of all the above, but because of their various handicaps cannot function fast enough or appropriately enough to participate in adequate turn taking. A person with a language processing problem, for instance, may digest information or formulate utterances too slowly to take part in a 'normal' fast moving taking of turns. Or, because of lowered self-esteem or insecurity, a communicatively handicapped person might regularly lose out when competing for overlapped turns or for turns in multiparty interactions.

Turn taking, like most other aspects of interaction, is influenced by social roles and motivations. In specific encounters not all participants have equal rights for taking and holding the floor. Again, this inequality is closely tied to who perceives themselves endowed with the right to control and impose. These rights might be attributed to one's professional obligation (e.g. teacher-pupil and clinician-client), to a long established social convention (e.g. woman-man and adult-child) or to individuals' self-perception of some kind of superiority (e.g. employer-employee). In such unequal encounters, the principles of turn taking are often suspended without negotiation and without explanation. Thus, for instance, men have been observed to talk, overlap and interrupt more than women in mixed-sex encounters, presumably reflecting men's feelings of superiority and women's feelings of inferiority (e.g. Zimmerman and West, 1975). This pattern is very similar to that between adults and children and, as was indicated above, between clinicians and clients (be they children or adults) in a structured therapy setting. Also, explicit turn allocation is a characteristic of unequal encounters where the person with more 'power' selects the next speaker turn, and in multi-party interactions the next speaker, by some such expressions or non-verbal cues as 'Say "fishing"', 'It's Paula next' or a nod in the direction of the next speaker. It may be that turns are allocated a great deal in 'traditional' clinical encounters, thus not enabling the client to practise turn dynamics which are characteristic of interactions beyond the clinical context.

Furthermore, the issue of whether clinical interactions provide adequate turn-taking models for clients needs to be considered. As was discussed above, in structured clinical interactions, turns tend to be allocated by clinicians (even in group therapy) thus diminishing the real-life pressures of competing for turns and repairing overlap. Clients also have no need to try to keep the floor since longer turns tend to be allowed in pre-allocated sequences (Sacks, Schegloff and Jefferson, 1974). Interrupting the clinician, even if appropriately, may not be looked upon favourably while the clinician has the right to interrupt the client without explanation. This is by no means to say that these behaviours occur in all clinical encounters but to highlight the potential, and often real, consequences because of the unbalanced nature of such interactions. Creating more communicatively relevant clinical interactions as part of one's therapy approach is a step towards more demanding, and potentially useful, turn dynamics (Chapter 7).

COHESION

One issue discourse analysis has addressed is how to describe the interrelatedness of thoughts and ideas in discourse and texts. One way of showing that meaning expressions are joined and linked to form coherent discourse is to look for linguistic indices in the actual surface text which serve the funtion of 'binding' the expressions together (see also coherence below). Such linguistic discourse markers have been extensively studied under the heading of 'cohesion' or 'cohesive devices'. A comprehensive overview of the cohesive devices in English is found in Halliday and Hasan (1976). Shorter overviews can be found in most introductory books on discourse analysis, notably de Beaugrande and Dressler (1981), Stubbs (1983) and Brown and Yule (1983). In this section, we shall first outline the main cohesive devices in English and then consider what value the identification of such devices may have for the speech-language clinician.

Quite often, but not always (see below), utterances are linked to one another via the meanings of words in one of the utterances being recoverable via reference to words in other utterances which have occurred either previously or are to occur subsequently. Consider the following two examples.

1. I saw my supervisor last week.
   She didn't have much to say.
2. This is what I told him.
   Never again will I let him decorate for me.

The meaning of the pronoun 'she' is recovered via reference to the previous utterance, the words 'my supervisor', and it is this referring back which binds the two utterances together; it is the semantic relation between the two items which renders the two utterances cohesive. 'She' can be referred to as a cohesive device or item and the link between 'she' and 'my supervisor' as a cohesive tie or a cohesive link. Similarly, in the second example the meaning of the word 'this' can be recovered via reference to the following utterance. In this case, it is the whole of the second utterance and the word 'this' which form a cohesive tie.

Cohesion in discourse is then created by listeners/text processors constantly linking utterances together by referring back and forth to what has been said (written) previously or will be said (written) subsequently. The term **anaphoric reference** or **anaphora** is used to describe those cohesive ties in which the meaning of the cohesive device is recovered via reference to **what has been before** (Halliday and Hasan, 1976). The first example above was one of anaphora. The second example illustrates **cataphoric reference** or **cataphora** in which relationship the meaning of the cohesive device is recovered via reference to **what is to follow** (Halliday and Hasan, 1976).

As exemplified thus far, cohesion is created by there being words in the discourse which are interpreted via reference to other words in that same discourse. And that this referring can be anaphoric or cataphoric in nature. The term **endophoric reference** is used to describe both referring backwards and forwards **within one piece of discourse** (Halliday and Hasan, 1976). This idea is contrasted with recovering meanings of cohesive devices via **reference to something in the extralinguistic context** (that is outside the spoken or written discourse itself). This is referred to as **exophoric reference** (Halliday and Hasan, 1976). In the following two examples the cohesive items are interpreted in reference to what is present in the physical context at the time of the expressions being uttered.

1. I love you.
2. Look at that.

In case of the first utterance there is likely to be no doubt who 'I' and 'you' refer to when uttered by one person to another. In the second example the real life referent of the cohesive item 'that' may be made apparent by accompanying pointing, head movement or gaze direction. The notion of exophoric reference describes the way all words in utterances gain meaning via reference outside the utterance and discourse itself. This might be via reference to something in the physical context, to something that has happened previously or is to happen in the future, to one's imaginary world and so on. In other words, all connecting of utterances in discourse happens within individual interpreters, and the cohesive markers (or, simply, words) serve as signposts for possible linking of expressions into a cohesive and coherent piece of discourse. Following Halliday and Hasan's model, exophoric reference differs from endophoric in that it is not cohesive in the sense of binding utterances together within one piece of discourse, rather it contributes towards the creation of cohesive discourse by linking the meaning expressions with the context of situation. Our main concern here is with cohesive devices within discourse (endophoric reference). Figure 3.1 summarizes the type of reference relationships discussed.

The term 'reference' has been used with two different meanings when discussing cohesion. Firstly, there is the general interpretation of cohesion created by referring back and forth within discourse. This refers to the simple instruction of 'see elsewhere' for the information which is required for the interpretation of the piece of discourse in question. Secondly, there is Halliday and Hasan's (1976) more specific meaning: the term 'reference' is used as a term for a specific type of referring within discourse which involves specific types of cohesive devices. In other words, in the former interpretation any cohesive device can enter a relationship of reference with any other item while in the latter instance only certain devices (e.g. pronouns, articles etc., see below) are said to enter this relationship. The

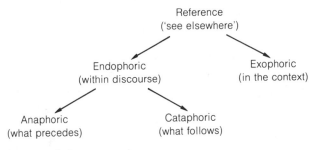

Fig. 3.1 Cohesive relations.

wider interpretation is all important for understanding how meaning expressions in discourse can be bound together, and the narrower meaning is useful for detailed description and understanding of the types of cohesive relationships in any one piece of discourse.

Halliday and Hasan outline five types of cohesive relationships and devices: Reference, Substitution, Ellipsis, Conjunction and Lexical Cohesion. Each of these will be briefly outlined and exemplified. For a much more detailed account the reader should refer to Halliday and Hasan (1976). Awareness of the type of cohesive devices promotes understanding of what discourse production and comprehension might involve.

The category 'Reference' consists of cohesive devices which are often referred to as grammatical, closed set items. More specifically, they are:

1. Personal pronouns (i.e. the forms I, you, she, he, it etc.; including 'one' and the forms mine, yours, his, ours etc.; including one's and my, your, his, our etc. and me, you, him, us etc.).
   e.g. Two men were standing close to one another. **One** said to the other: 'I will never forget what **you** have done for **me**'.
2. Demonstrative pronouns (i.e. this, that, these, those, here, there).
   e.g. A. We went to the Steak House last night.
        B. **That** must have been quite an occasion.
   e.g. A. Devon is one of my favourite places.
        B. Yes. It's beautiful **there**.
   e.g. A. First he broke the window and then he managed to break the windowsill!
        B. **That** boy is unbelievable.
3. The definite article 'the'.
   e.g. Once upon a time there was a beautiful princess. But **the** princess was very lonely.
4. Comparative forms expressing likeness or unlikeness between things (e.g. words such as same, equal, identical, similar, such, so, other, different, otherwise etc.)
   e.g. A. The car had a dent in the bumper.
        B. I must have seen **the same** car.

e.g. A. It has blue patterns on a green background.
     B. Mine is quite **different**.

The first three are more readily identifiable and are the ones most often applied to the study of communication handicaps (Chapters 5 and 6). Also, the above personal and demonstrative forms are often referred to as **deictic** expressions (or **deixis**), meaning that their interpretation is dependent on either the co-occurring utterances or the wider context. As such deixis extends beyond the above reference items to many other semantically 'empty' words (e.g. 'thing'; 'stuff') which acquire meaning via reference to other items or context (e.g. substitute items, below). Levinson (1983) provides an accessible discussion on deixis (person, time, space, discourse and social).

    Substitution, as the second type of cohesive relationship, describes the replacement of one word by another. Indeed, this is how reference could be defined too. Let us first consider the different types of substitution devices and then explore how Halliday and Hasan differentiate substitution from reference. To avoid repetition of words in discourse, the subsequent occurrence of the word can be replaced by substitutes. Substitutes can be categorized into nominal, verbal and clausal ones. This reflects the grammatical functions of the substitutes: a noun, a verb or a clause. The following is a list of words which can function as one of these substitutes.

1. Nominal: a noun phrase, either only the head or the head plus the modifiers, is replaced by 'one', 'ones' or 'the same'.
   e.g. A. Which flower would you like?
       B. I want that **one** (flower = a noun/the head).
   e.g. A. A campari and soda, please.
       B. I'll have **the same**. (a campari and soda = the whole noun phrase).
2. Verbal: a verb phrase, often an extended one including complements, is replaced by 'do' in the appropriate morphological form.
   e.g. A. Did Peter seem very unwell?
       B. Not really. But, Alison **did** (seemed very unwell = an extended verb group).

   e.g. A. Did he leave the keys?
        B. He **should have done** (should have left the keys).
3. Clausal: an entire clause is replaced by 'so' or 'not'.
   e.g. A. I wonder if there is going to be a thunderstorm?
        B. I believe **so** (that there is going to be a thunderstorm).
   e.g. A. Are they going to invite the Smiths?
        B. I hope **not** (that they are not going to invite the Smiths).

The question is then how substitution differs from reference. As we have seen from the above examples, the same lexical items, namely 'one', 'so' and 'the same', can in fact enter both cohesive relations. Halliday and Hasan give several criteria for differentiating between the two (Halliday and Hasan 1976, 88–90, 142–146). The most workable approach concerns the relationship between the cohesive item and item(s) it refers to. When two items enter the relation of reference, they refer to exactly the same idea or entity in the real world. With substitution, this relationship is not however identical but some additional specification is added to the definition of the substitute. To illustrate this, let us reconsider the above examples for the lexical item 'one' in both of the relationships.

1. Reference
   e.g. Two men were standing close to one another. **One** said to the other . . .

Here the cohesive item 'one' refers to one of the two men. It does not imply any additional specification of which men the reference is to.

2. Substitution
   e.g. A. Which flower would you like?
        B. I want **that one**.

Here the cohesive item 'one' does not refer to exactly the same concept of 'flower' as the word 'flower' it refers to. As signalled by the determiner 'that' the word 'one' has a narrower meaning than the original word.

The third type of cohesive relationship, ellipsis, can be defined as substitution by zero. What this means is that something is left unsaid but is implied and the meaning of this implication is recoverable from what has been said or written before. The items which are not expressed but are implied can be noun phrases, verb phrases or parts of clauses, and thus we refer to nominal, verbal and clausal ellipsis. As is apparent from the examples (2) below, verbal ellipsis involves absence of other clausal elements than verbs alone.

1. Nominal:
   e.g. A. Could I have some wine please?
   B. Sorry. There isn't any (**wine** = a noun).
2. Verbal/Clausal:
   e.g. A. You haven't taken your tablets today.
   B. Yes I have (**taken my tablets today** = the main verb, a noun and an adverb ellipsed).
   A. Are you reading?
   B. No.
   Writing (**I am** = an auxiliary verb and a pronoun ellipsed).

Conjunction, the fourth type of cohesive relationship, is somewhat different from the others discussed so far. Reference, substitution and ellipsis bind expressions together by one having to refer back (and sometimes forth) for interpretation of the current expression. While cohesive chains are often formed over longer stretches of discourse, the relationship between a cohesive item and the item it refers to is one-to-one. It is, so to speak, a fairly local relationship. Conjunctions as cohesive devices, on the other hand, do not require any anaphoric or cataphoric referring for their interpretation. They create cohesion by virtue of their inherent meaning which in turn binds together bigger chunks of discourse. It is a more global cohesive device than the others. Conjunctions, such as 'or', 'but' 'in other words' and 'on the other hand', function as processing facilitators for the listener/text receiver, indicating how whole ideas in discourse relate to one another beyond the relatedness of individual lexical items.

There are many possible meaning relationships within discourse and consequently many conjunctions which can serve to indicate them. Conjunctions are those words or phrasal expressions which have the above kind of cohesive

function. Halliday and Hasan classify conjunctive relations
into four main types: additive, adversative, causal and
temporal (Halliday and Hasan, 1976, 226–273).

1. Additive: Additive conjunctions indicate that what is
   to follow simply provides additional information to
   what has already been given. This information can highlight similarity or dissimilarity between the previous
   information and what is to follow. Conjunctions such as
   'and', 'or', 'furthermore', 'in addition', 'that is', 'for
   instance', 'thus', 'similarly' and 'on the other hand'
   serve as examples of additive relations. What needs
   to be noted is that some of these conjunctions (notably,
   'and' and 'or'), and others discussed below, may also
   bind together clauses within utterances. Such use of
   conjunction does not contribute towards creating cohesive discourse as discussed here.
2. Adversative: Adversative conjunctions convey the basic
   meaning that what is to follow is contrary to expectation.
   This expectation may reflect not only what has been
   expressed previously but also what is expected in the
   speaker-listener relationship, or in the communicative
   context as a whole. Examples of adversative conjunctions
   are: 'but', 'yet', 'actually', 'however', 'on the other hand',
   'rather' and 'on the contrary'.
3. Causal: Causal conjunctions imply relations such as
   cause–effect, result and purpose. Conjunctions such
   as 'so', 'therefore', 'because', 'consequently', 'for this
   reason', 'as a result', 'with this in mind', 'in this regard',
   'with reference to' and 'in that case' serve a causal
   function.
4. Temporal: Temporal conjunctions express the meaning
   of one event ᴖᴄcurring at a different time from another.
   The 'event' may be something that actually happens
   in real time or it can be a sequence of points made in
   written discourse. The following are examples of temporal conjunctions: 'then', 'next', 'previously', 'finally',
   'an hour later', 'meanwhile', 'up to now, 'briefly' and
   'to sum up'.

The fifth, and final, cohesive relation discussed in Halliday
and Hasan is that of lexical cohesion. This is yet again dif-

ferent from all the others. Lexical cohesion is created in discourse by virtue of words being semantically related to one another. That is to say that words about the same topic, part of the same semantic fields, form cohesive links across discourse. Halliday and Hasan distinguish between two types of lexical cohesion; reiteration and collocation.

1. Reiteration: Cohesion is created by repetition of the same lexical item, by use of a more general or specific term, by use of synonyms, near-synonyms, superordinates or any words which the listener perceives as 'being about the same topic'.

2. Collocation: This refers to the creation of cohesion via lexical items that regularly co-occur. This mainly refers to lexical relations such as antonomy (oppositeness) and hyponomy (meaning inclusion) and words that are part of (ordered) sets such as days of the week, the spectrum of colour and the monetary system.

Having now outlined the main types of cohesive relations, it needs to be emphasized that analysing discourse with these categories is not always straightforward. There is some overlap between the categories: as already pointed out above the distinction between reference and substitution may not always be clear. Similarly, there has been discussion where deictic 'empty' expressions such as 'thing(y)', 'whatsitsname' and 'stuff' fit in. Like reference items and substitutes they also gain their meaning via reference to something in the context or the co-text. Yet, from the linguistic point of view they are more like lexical items than grammatical forms. While it is not particularly relevant for a practising clinician to enter such a linguistic debate, it is nevertheless important to recognize the similarity between these lexical items and the other deictic items discussed under the relation of reference.

What a speech-language clinician might be asking now is whether the distinctions between the different types of cohesive relationships are particularly relevant for a practising professional, or do they simply reflect theoretical distinctions in a linguistic taxonomy? In other words, how could description of a client's discourse in terms of cohesion aid our understanding of the client as a communicator?

We shall address these issues in some detail in Chapter 4, where discourse analysis based on cohesion is used as an example of how a discourse framework for analysis might function. We shall simply note here that analysis of cohesion can tell us about the client's ability to presuppose what their interlocutor can process, their ability to link ideas some distance apart, their notion of redundancy in discourse and their range and distribution of vocabulary. It may also be that a sense of self, linked to a sense of the similarity of other people to oneself, is required in order to handle these discourse skills. If this is the case, the suggestion that certain people may lack a 'theory of mind' (Baron-Cohen, Leslie and Frith, 1985) is relevant. It was suggested that conditions such as autism might involve inability to appreciate or even imagine the mental processes of other people. The use of deixis by such individuals is one of the major sources of data for this hypothesis (e.g. Jordan, 1989).

COHERENCE

Discourse is about linking of ideas and thoughts together to express emotions, to initiate action, to maintain relationships and so on. As we saw above, discourse is said to be cohesive when there are linguistic markers in the surface text which indicate that the expressions are linked. Yet, cohesive discourse does not guarantee that the thoughts and ideas are linked (make sense) for the listener. Consider the following extract from an answer by a schizophrenic adult to the question 'How did you come to be in the hospital?' (Gordon, 1990).

> 'Somebody called Cliff Richard. He seems to project my image back to him. Whether he was born at the same time and I'm a twin of his is debatable. Because we have gone through quite a lot of things together over the years that have been quite extraordinary to me.'

We can identify many cohesive links between the utterances (e.g. Cliff Richard – he – him – he – his – we – together). Indeed, this stretch of discourse is in many respects cohesive even though problems with cohesion also exist (e.g.

use of 'because'). The main problem is however that this extract does not really answer the original question and that the listener cannot readily (if at all) identify what the topic under discussion is and how it is developed. The discourse notion of coherence enables one to investigate such problems in topical development. The term coherence can be taken to refer to the interrelatedness of senses, thoughts and ideas underneath the surface of the discourse (e.g. de Beaugrande and Dressler, 1981). There are many texts on coherence which examine the notion of coherence in great detail. The following provide accessible and thorough accounts of the notion: de Beaugrande and Dressler, 1981; Brown and Yule, 1983; Craig and Tracy, 1983; MacLaughlin, 1984.

Coherence is a complex phenomenon to analyse reflecting such basic difficulties as what is meant by sense, thoughts and ideas. Furthermore, creating continuity of senses in discourse involves inferencing and active problem solving which in turn are listener/text receiver specific. A psychiatrist, a nurse, a relative, a language specialist or someone with no experience with mental disorders would probably interpret the above extract differently. The role of inferencing is central for creating coherence in discourse. By inferencing we mean making connections between ideas in discourse. At one extreme there may be no apparent surface clues as to the interrelatedness of ideas, and yet by reference to human knowledge and experience connections can be made. Consider the following interchange:

A. Will you attend tomorrow?
B. My mother is not too well.

While there is nothing in the actual words themselves which connects B's utterance to A's, we can, without any difficulty, interpret B's utterance as a negative answer. All communication is based on active inferencing on the part of the listener, the extent of which being dependent on our familiarity with the world which is being discussed and on the explicit signalling of how utterances are intended to be connected. When explicitly signalling discourse connections by means of cohesive devices one needs to strike a balance between too explicit, and potentially boring, and not explicit enough, and thus potentially obscure (de Beaugrande and Dressler, 1981). There are of course instances where one tries to minimize inferencing by maximizing explicitness (e.g. fire instructions) or vice versa (e.g. when trying to mislead; when creating literary allusion or poetic effect).

The notion of coherence can be approached from the angle that any discourse, be it written or spoken, can be described in terms of sequences of topics. While on the surface this appears a fairly workable descriptive approach, it presents one very big problem: How do we identify a topical unit? In simple terms, a topic is what is being talked about. In any extended piece of discourse there are likely to be several larger 'discourse topics' and smaller sub-topics which are related to and develop the discourse topics (Brown and Yule, 1983). For instance, talking about one's holiday (discourse topic) could consist of such sub-topics as 'getting there', 'accommodation', 'surroundings', 'what we did' and 'the friends we made'. In this way, topic is defined in terms of the semantic relatedness of the content of utterances. This definition can, however, pose several problems. As was discussed above, a discourse topic or a sub-topic does not necessarily coincide with different speakers' perception of semantic units within discourse (see speaker's topic; Brown and Yule, 1983, 87–94). While there is likely to be agreement amongst people who share life experiences and values as to what is being talked/written about at any one time, it is not uncommon to have idiosyncratic interpretations, which potentially affect one's perception of the incidence and frequency of topical units. Secondly, it is not always apparent where one topic ends and another begins when topics are closely related. In fact, how far apart conceptually do topics need to be for one to identify them as separate topics? On similar lines, what is the nature of the relationship between discourse topics and sub-topics in terms of semantic relatedness? There are no answers to these questions, since people's intuitions are difficult to formalize. Also, the creation and development of topics are speaker and genre specific. The fluidity of topics by people suffering from schizophrenia contrasts sharply with an even less predictable informal chat between 'normally functioning' individuals.

Rather than trying to undertake the difficult task of providing a definition of what a topic is, it may be more useful to try to determine topical boundary markers (Brown and Yule, 1983). In other words, bearing in mind the problems indicated in the previous paragraph, we look for linguistic markers which serve to indicate topic change or shift. Again, while such markers are ultimately genre specific, we all recognize adverbial connectors such as 'firstly', 'secondly', 'finally', 'on the other hand' and 'however' as indices of shift in (sub)topic (see also cohesion above). Similarly, phrases such as 'Let me make another point', 'To take a different view . . .' and 'Consider also' function as introductions to new (sub)topics (see also metacommunication above). Being able to change and to perceive the change of topics appropriately by using boundary markers is a complex pragmatic skill (Chapters 1 and 5).

Paragraphs in written texts can also function as topical boundary markers (Longacre, 1979; Brown and Yule, 1983) even though one topic or subtopic can be developed in more than one paragraph. Paragraph divisions may be motivated not only by topical chunks but also by stylistic appeal or printing conventions. Similarly, spoken language has also its means of signalling new topics. By intonational variation, phonological prominance and raised pitch the beginning of a new topic can be signalled (Brown and Yule, 1983). Similarly, the end of a spoken topic can be indicated by low pitch, reduced loudness and a pause (cf. Sacks *et al.*, 1974; end of turn signals; also turn taking above).

Bearing in mind the apparently indeterminate nature of the notion of topic and the resulting problems for the notion of coherence in discourse, people do nevertheless identify topics and subtopics in discourse and accordingly can make relevant and appropriate contributions which can develop topics further, change the focus of topics or initiate altogether new topics. There must be some intuitive agreement amongst language users that a topic has certain semantic unity amongst its constituent parts (expressions). This semantic unity forms, however, a continuum from totally related expressions to those that are loosely connected via often quite idiosyncratic inferencing.

The concept of coherence is a relevant one for the understanding of communication problems. It can provide a means of focusing on irrelevance, topical drifting, lack of elaboration and the types of semantic relationships holding between ideas. Examining coherence in discourse also enables one to explore why listeners may find it difficult to process particular pieces of discourse (e.g. Gordon, 1990). We shall first examine an analytical framework developed for the analysis of foreign learner compositions (Leinonen-Davies, 1984, 1988b) and then consider its applicability to the clinical context. While this is a framework for analysing written texts or spoken monologues, much of it is applicable to the analysis of dialogues. Space does not allow us to give adequate emphasis to both monologues and dialogues, and thus we shall not consider the latter in any detail here.

The basic idea of this framework comes from de Beaugrande and Dressler's (1983) notion of coherence networks. We can begin with the idea that in coherent pieces of discourse all expressions, or propositions if we focus on their semantic content, are related to one another in some way and to a discourse topic or a sub-topic. If we imagine a story with a title, we expect all the propositions in that story to be about the topic specified by the title. We also expect all the sub-topics to be related to the topic. But this is not enough for a story to be coherent. We also expect the propositions to develop the story towards some prespecified goal(s), one(s) most likely specified by the title. Producing discourse is generally goal-oriented behaviour. Excepting occasions when one 'drifts' when talking about a topic one knows very little about or when tired, drunk or otherwise mentally incapable, one generally tries to get somewhere, tries to make a point. And when developing a topic, in written discourse at least, those aspects of the topic which serve to make a particular point follow one another in sequence. While this is a likely aim in spoken discourse as well, the time pressure of formulating propositions on one's feet regularly makes one add and amend previously developed topics ('Could I just go back to X? Oh, and there is this other thing . . .'). Within this background, four types of coherence in discourse can be identified.

1. Propositions expressed in discourse are related to a discourse topic and/or sub-topics. This can be referred to as **propositional coherence**.
2. Propositions developing the same topic or sub-topic are in some semantic/logical relationship to one another. This can be referred to as **relational coherence**.
3. Propositions develop a topic or a sub-topic towards a specified goal. This can be referred to as **rhetorical coherence**.
4. Those propositions which describe closely related aspects of a discourse topic or a sub-topic follow one another in sequence. This can be referred to as **sequential coherence**.

These four aspects of coherence by no means constitute an exhaustive account of what coherence entails. For practical purposes, however, they allow one to systematize some of those familiar hunches we all have about incoherent and coherent pieces of discourse. They enable one to examine topical development, and what might have gone wrong with it.

If these four types of coherence capture some of the features of coherent texts, then by implication, incoherent texts can be characterized by:

1. Propositions which are not related to the discourse topic or sub-topics;
2. Propositions which are not related to one another;
3. Propositions which do not develop the topic/sub-topic towards a goal and;
4. Semantically closely related propositions which do not follow one another in sequence.

These, in turn, can be related to such familiar feelings as:

1. Not knowing how to relate what is currently being talked about to what is generally being talked about;
2. Finding it difficult to see how ideas are related to one another;
3. Feeling the speaker/writer, while still talking about the same topic, has gone off at a tangent; and
4. Finding the speaker/writer is changing back and forth between topics.

By such initial feelings we often identify that something has gone amiss. To be able to do something constructive about these feelings we need to be able to pinpoint more precisely what it might be in the client's behaviour which contributes towards these feelings of dissatisfaction. The above types of coherence provide a means of exploring these issues in a principled manner.

To be able to examine coherence or incoherence in discourse, it is helpful to establish some kind of graphic mode of representation of the way propositions are related to one another and to the discourse topic. While several approaches are viable, we find it most descriptive to actually draw a diagram representing coherence in specific texts. While such representation is time-consuming, especially when dealing with very incoherent pieces of discourse, it is worthwhile for its clarity and subsequent usefulness. Also, as one becomes more competent with examining incoherence in discourse, one can develop less demanding methods of description. Yet, initially, drawing diagrams is a very educational enterprise. It helps one to appreciate the complex and at times intangible nature of the interrelatedness of ideas in discourse.

For the sake of clarity, let us consider a diagram which represents the development of one topic only. And let us call that the discourse topic and assume that it is the above mentioned question 'How did you come to be in the hospital?'. And let us assume that we are analysing the

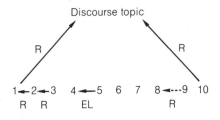

R = Reason
EL = Elaboration

Fig. 3.2 Coherence relationships

following reconstructed text from answers by schizophrenic adults (Gorden, 1990), reconstructed in order to capture as many key points as possible in a short extract.

1. I came here to recuperate.
2. I had a nervous breakdown.
3. I couldn't cope with anything.
4. I think about things.
5. I think about the names Paige and Rice.
6. P-a-i-g-e is a p-a-g-e in a book.
7. P-a-i-g-e becomes p-a-g-e to me.
8. I like going around my mum's house a lot.
9. I tried to make amends with my dad.
10. My problem is that I don't make the same connections like you can.

In order to investigate propositional coherence, the discourse topic is placed in such a position in the diagram that it allows one to relate all the propositions to it directly if such a direct relationship exists (Figure 3.2). Then each of the propositions in the text is numbered and related to the discourse topic and to one another, if such relatedness exists. Arrows are drawn to link the propositions together. A solid arrow indicates a fairly direct relationship while a broken arrow indicates a less direct one. The 'directness' reflects the amount of inferencing one needs to carry out to arrive at a link (see above). The extent of inferencing in turn may reflect the extent of explicit signalling of cohesion in the surface text: the more explicit the signalling, the less inferencing needed, provided the listener is familiar with the subject matter. Further dimensions can be added to the representation, which however will not be discussed here, since the text under discussion does not require these further devices (Leinonen-Davies, 1984, 1988b).

While the notations elucidated so far enable one to examine the four types of coherence, to gain additional relevant information about topical development, we can specify the nature of the semantic relatedness of the propositions. Following some such notation as Sorensen's (1981) (Leinonen-Davies, 1984, 1988b) one proposition can be seen in relationships such as 'reason of', 'elaboration of' and 'concretizaton of' in relation to other propositions.

Within this background, let us briefly examine Figure 3.2 which represents the above piece of discourse. As can be seen, only the propositions 1, 2, 3 and 10 are directly about the discourse topic (as perceived by the current authors). 2 and 3 specify 1 further by adding information. Proposition 4 could be perceived as another reason for this person being in hospital, in particular in view of our knowledge that the speaker suffers from schizophrenia which in turn can indicate a thought disorder. Within this premise, proposition 5 can be thought of as specifying 4 further. It is however quite impossible to relate 6 and 7 to anything. 8 and 9, while not being related to the discourse topic, form a pocket of coherence within an otherwise incoherent stretch of text. And then 10 functions as a kind of summary, being related to the topic.

Having examined the specific characteristics of this piece of discourse, it can then be discussed in more general terms, relating the discussion to the four types of coherence. Reflecting the lack of links between the propositions and the discourse topic the text is largely propositionally incoherent. The text is first about the topic, but because of the apparently uninterpretable utterances (4,5,6,7) and their apparent non-connectedness to anything else the text receiver cannot make the necessary links. As such, the text can also be said to be largely relationally incoherent (i.e. the ideas within seem largely unconnected). Nothing can be said about rhetorical and sequential incoherence in relation to this small sample.

The above description pinpoints where the client is encountering problems. He/she appears to have problems with:

1. Talking about a topic beyond a few utterances;
2. Signalling explicitly to the listener how utterances are related;
3. Developing a topic towards a goal.

By interrelating these 'symptoms' with diagnostic categories it may be possible to arrive at a diagnosis. What use this would be for the actual management of the problem is not however clear. A more meaningful approach might consider what the client would need to be able to do to remedy the situation. By asking this question, we aim to explore the underlying abilities necessary for the production of coherent discourse (Chapter 4). In this instance, the client would need to be able to:

1. Identify a topic and the goal specified by it;
2. Identify what is relevant and irrelevant to this topic;
3. Identify which of the relevant aspects are about the same topic;
4. Order the relevant aspects.

At another level, we might ask what the client would need to be able to do to be able to do 1–4. This would involve delving into the prerequisites for producing language and discourse at all (Chapter 1). Such explorations would then feed directly into treatment plans.

Accepting all this, a clinician may still ask whether there is any particular need to carry out a detailed analysis such as the above. It depends on how observant, experienced and familiar with discourse concepts any individual clinician is. Yet, even if one could easily identify many of the problems leading to incoherence without a detailed account, description can help to identify such very specific features as islands of meaning within an otherwise incomprehensible passage, relatedness or unrelatedness of ideas which were not apparent when simply listening to the piece and other such features which can go undetected solely because of the impossibility of handling complex networks in one's mind. On the other hand, one readily recognizes the common lack of time for detailed analysis in the clinical context. Accepting this, familiarity with detailed analysis, even if not used as a regular analytical tool, can heighten one's powers of observation and can lead to meaningful remedial programmes.

INFORMATIVITY

Discourse is also a carrier of information. The notion of informativity in discourse can be explored from two main perspectives:

1. The extent to which a given message is expected or unexpected.

2. The manner in which information is structured within discourse.

We shall examine each in turn and shall refer the reader to additional information in de Beaugrande and Dressler (1981), Halliday (1967, 1968) and Danes (1974).

The idea that messages carry a certain amount of information derives from a mathematical theory of communication, called Information Theory, which was devised to maximize the efficiency of signal transmission in telecommunications (Shannon and Weaver, 1949, Miller, 1951, Lyons, 1977). It serves our purpose here simply to note the principle of statistical probability of occurrence. In short, the greater the probability of occurrence of a signal, the less information it contains. Thus, if a signal is totally predictable, it carries no information. As such, information is tied to the notions of predictability and redundancy and, consequently, to what the listener requires to hear to be able to process a message. It is well known that language expressions carry a certain amount of redundancy. One can communicate without many grammatical function words. Pidgin and creole languages, the language of children, foreign language learners and the communicatively handicapped may employ mainly content words, and the grammatical relations which hold between them can be inferred by reference to the structure of the language, the content of the words present and the communicative context (e.g. (the) Puppet is (in the) box). In the sense of information theory, information is tied solely to the notion of probability of occurrence of items. It is a useful notion for anyone who encounters structurally incomplete utterances. Structural incompleteness does not necessarily imply lack of informativity in utterances because of predictability and redundancy in human communication systems.

The notion of informativity has other facets to it, which are also of interest to those dealing with communication problems. Expressions can be said to be informative if they are new or unexpected to the receivers de Beaugrande and Dressler, 1981; Lyons, 1977). By 'new' we mean making the receiver aware of something which he/she was not aware of previously. As such informativity is closely tied to the background knowledge of the participants. The notion of unexpectedness encompasses this idea of newness plus the idea of something being informative via being surprising and therefore interesting. Whereas the notion of unexpectedness is generally applied to the content of meaning expressions, elements of any aspect of the language system can be informative in the sense of being surprising. Putting on a funny voice, speaking with a foreign accent, clapping one's hands unexpectedly or using an unusual syntactic pattern (e.g. poetry) can render expressions interesting and/or challenging to process, and thus more informative. There must, however, be a threshold for each individual where non-ordinariness becomes disturbing, and thus potentially non-communicative. Being aware in the clinical context that communication is based on these notions of informativeness enables one to re-evaluate the informativity of clinical interactions and to address the question to what extent should and can clinical interactions adhere to the principles of informativeness. Is it one of the goals of such interactions to be informative? Does being informative aid or hinder learning of skill?

One of the tasks speakers undertake when formulating meaning expressions is to try to determine what the listener knows and does not know about the world, what is new or old information to the listener (Chapter 1). In doing so, speakers try to pitch 'the right' level of information in their message. What this right level may be depends entirely on each participant's background knowledge and their shared knowledge. Clearly, determining what one's interlocutor's life experiences might or might not have been is a complex piecing together of any available information, ranging from long-standing knowledge of the other's life, values and beliefs to forming impressions on the basis of appearance, speech, occupation or almost any clue. The speaker can also rely on many metacommunicative statements to check whether his/her hypotheses were accurate, in order not to presuppose too much or too little ('Did you know about X?'; 'You probably know that . . .'). From the listener's perspective, striking a balance between too obvious or not obvious enough affects the processing of the information. If a message is largely old information, a listener may find it difficult to maintain interest and thus may stop listening. On the other hand, if a message contains too much new information the listener may not be able to relate it to existing knowledge frames for interpretation, and again may stop listening. It is easy to feel bored, overwhelmed, disinterested or annoyed when one's interlocutors have failed to strike the balance. When checking during interactions whether one's interactants do find the current topics interesting and worthwhile, one needs to strike a balance between self respect and respect for others. What this ultimately comes down to is the avoidance of pseudo-coversations which do not matter to anybody. Such conversations are common in clinical interactions. Asking an adult mentally handicapped person what the colour of his shirt is or what he had for breakfast are topics which reflect minimal respect for oneself and for one's interactive partner. And the information content of such utterances is non-existent. They do, however, carry much meaning: 'I don't know how to handle this situation'; 'I am not interested in this interaction'; 'It is my duty to say something' or 'I believe this is all the other person can process'. Avoiding pseudo-conversations does not however imply the avoidance of small talk which keeps the communicative channel open. One becomes worried, however, if the main bulk of conversational interaction consists of such channel openers.

The other main aspect of discourse which can be discussed under informativity concerns how information is structured within a piece of discourse itself. The above notions hinge upon how speakers and listeners find pieces of discourse in terms of the newness, unexpectedness and predictability of the form and content of the expressions. Each expression within discourse can also be said to carry new or old information in relation to what has been expressed in the actual discourse previously. This is not tied to speakers' or listeners' knowledge but to what has previously occurred. Thus, each expression can be thought of as having a 'given' and a 'new' component to it; the given implying what has been mentioned previously and the 'new' what has not been mentioned previously. See also Danes (1974) who uses the term 'theme' for given and 'rheme' for new. Indeed, stating that expressions have a given or a new component is a means of describing how expressions develop to form larger pieces of discourse. The terms 'known' and 'unknown' have also been used in the context of informativity (Halliday, 1967, 1968). They do not correspond to the notions of given/theme (known) and new/ rheme (unknown). Known and unknown refer to the idea of listeners being aware or unaware of the content of utterances (i.e. to the first mentioned notion of informativity).

Let us consider a short extract from a conversation between a ten-year-old 'pragmatically' dysfunctioning boy, Simon, and his therapist. Simon is telling a story while looking at a book he is familiar with but the therapist is not. Nor can the therapist see the pictures in the book.

S. Puts his hat on.
   Rides a bike.
T. Who does?
S. The gorilla.
T. Oh. I see.
S. Rides in the road.
   Has a sweep.
T. He's trying to clear up all the mess he's made.
S. Puts a bucket on his head.
   The boy tips some water on his head.

Using a syntactic framework of analysis, Simon's utterances can be said to be lacking the subject. A remedial programme might then focus on sentential subjects. Describing the utterances in this way, we concentrate solely on the individual utterances, and do not consider what the consequences of the lack of subjects are for the discourse as a whole. Within a discourse framework, Simon's utterances can be described as lacking the given or themes; that is the information which relates the utterances to previous utterances (in addition to some possible problems in cohesive use of pronouns). And consequently, it is difficult for the therapist to follow how the topic is being developed. Some of the utterances can also be described in terms of violating the known/unknown distinction. When the missing theme corresponds to the known then no problem arises for the listener (i.e. the listener can recover the missing information elsewhere). But when the missing theme corresponds to the unknown then a problem of recoverability is likely to result. So, from the point of view of the communicative adequacy of utterances, it is more meaningful to describe individual utterances in terms of their information structures than some abstract grammatical structures such as subject, predicate and object. In this way, it is possible to examine the consequences incomplete utterances may have on the development of topics within discourse (see coherence above) and the interpretability of utterances by the listeners. Missing grammatical subjects might have no effect on communicating meanings and thus introduction of subjects into a client's grammatical 'system' would not be a top priority for someone who is failing as a communicator of meanings.

A final point we wish to consider in this section stems from the idea of discourse information structure. What are worth considering are the motivations for ascribing certain information to the theme/given slot and certain information to the rheme/new slot. Since the theme represents the information previously mentioned, then what occupies the theme slot is determined by previously mentioned information. But how do we decide what goes in the first theme slot? Speakers/text producers want to present their information from a certain perspective and accordingly choose the theme of the first utterance to set up this perspective. The perspective is set up by each new topic within any piece of discourse. It is for this reason that syntactic structure is textually and communicatively motivated. It is the discourse or topic perspective which determines, for instance, whether an active or a passive construction is appropriate or whether one chooses such a marked syntactic structure such as 'it was X that . . .'. If we consider the following two sentences

1. Jenny provided the costumes.
2. The costumes were provided by Jenny.

the active sentence (1) can be perceived as focusing on 'what Jenny did' while the passive sentence (2) focuses on 'how the costumes were acquired'. Syntactic structures are motivated by discourse consideration and by the theme we direct the interpretation of the utterance by setting up the perspective from which to process the new information in the rheme slot. We may question the value of teaching syntactic structure separated from the discourse context it serves. Since language is for communication, it may not prove workable to separate structure from its function for too long. A temporary separation may however assist diagnosis and remediation to some extent.

COMMUNICATION STRATEGIES

The final aspect of communication we wish to examine in this section concerns some ways in which all communicators in general, and those who find communication problematic in particular, try to overcome problems by employing certain strategies. By the word 'strategy' we mean behaviour which is designed to deal with a problem. The issue of how consciously or subconsciously strategies are employed will not be pursued here. What one needs to recognize is that strategies may be more or less conscious or subconscious and that this has implications for the management of communication problems.

Being at a loss for a word, we may talk about the characteristics of the entity ('It's a bit like an orange but a bit yellower'), we may change our goal midstream ('I frequently . . . I see my relatives all the time') or abandon the topic altogether. By employing any of these methods, we recognize (consciously or subconsciously) that a problem exists and deal with it by whatever means we have available at that time and/or by means which are appropriate for the specific problem. The concept of communication strategy (CS) was introduced in the foreign language learning context to capture some of the means by which learners deal with gaps in their linguistic competence to achieve communicative goals (Selinker, 1972, Tarone, Cohen and Dumas, 1976, Tarone, 1983, Faerch and Kasper, 1983). The notion of CS shifted focus from considering non-native-like expressions as mere indices of inadequate command of the target language (i.e. errors) to viewing them as positive indicators of the learner actively coping with communicative demands. A communicatively handicapped individual is clearly in a similar position to the second language learner:

he or she may lack the means of producing target language expressions and consequently may resort to a CS to solve or minimize the problem. Given that there does appear to be this parallel, it becomes crucial to determine whether, or to what extent, an apparently disabled communicator has available the language knowledge and ability to produce correct forms. Some may possess the means but lack confidence, thus resorting to less demanding CSs. Some may lack the means but have awareness and ability with regard to possible CSs. Others may lack both the means and awareness of, or ability to use, CS to alleviate communication problems. Being aware of these different possibilities enables one to differentiate between those who may have a pragmatically based problem of not being aware of CS and those who are aware but cannot resort to them because they lack the means of resorting to, or the confidence to resort to, CSs (Chapter 5).

We shall first outline the theoretical concept of CSs and then consider how it has been, and can be, applied to the speech pathology context. We shall concentrate on the Faerch-Kasper (1983) model of CSs here. Within this framework, CSs are explored within a model of speech production. CSs can also be receptive in nature (i.e. a person may devise strategies for dealing with comprehension problems), but these are much less accessible for study, and consequently are less understood. One example would be one pausing to allow time for processing before responding. We shall concentrate on productive/expressive strategies only and on those which manifest themselves as a consequence of a problem in producing language.

Faerch and Kasper start with the premise that communication is largely goal oriented and that achieving this goal involves planning and subsequent execution of the plan. A problem may arise at the planning or the execution stages in that the person does not have the specific language expression available (for whatever reason) or may not be able to execute it. When encountering this problem, the person has several choices. He or she may abandon the overall communicative goal altogether, may modify the goal or may retain the overall goal but change the specific plan. To take an example, a person may wish to ask another person what the best way to get from A to B is (overall communicative goal). Let us assume that the person with this goal tends to stutter and experiences difficulty in executing the specific utterance. When experiencing this difficulty the person can decide:

1. Not to ask for the directions after all, but rather carry on studying the map (abandon the communicative goal);
2. To ask where A is on the map (modify the communicative goal);
3. To ask for directions by pointing to A and B on the map (retain the goal but change the plan).

By engaging in any of the activities in (1)–(3), the person can be said to be employing a CS. The person is somehow trying to cope with the problem.

There is one crucial aspect of communication which is not taken into account in this example based on the Faerch-Kasper model of CSs. The over-all communicative goal is motivated by a personal goal of wanting in the first instance to get from A to B. For one to have any need to formulate the communicative goal of asking for directions one has to have the need to know the specific route. In other words, communicative behaviours are driven by personal goals which are significant for individual communicators. When experiencing difficulty with executing an utterance to achieve the personal and communicative goals in the above example, the person has also the option of

4. Not wanting to (or convincing oneself that one does not want to) get from A to B (abandoning the personal goal).

This option can have the most detrimental consequences not only for the person as a communicator but also as a human being. Compromising one's personal goals can undermine one's self-esteem and confidence and can isolate one from human interaction. It is a drastic option indicating that the person is not coping with the problem, rather than trying to resort to strategies to solve the problem one chooses to igore it. Opting out is, however, a legitimate pragmatic strategy and every person has the right to resort to it if they so wish. As a speech-language professional, one needs to be able to determine whether opting out has

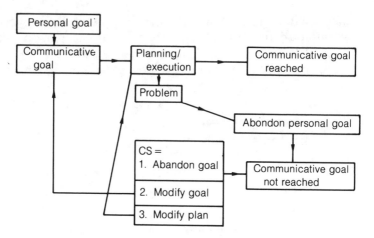

Fig. 3.3 CS in the speech production model.

positive or negative implications for the person's mental and physical well-being. The notion of a personal goal in communication has many implications for the management of communication disorders as well. For instance, it questions assessment and treatment based on activities with no real significance for the communicators and it draws one's attention to potentially inappropriate labelling of the absence of communicative behaviours as indices of lack of communicative ability.

The place of CSs within the model of speech production is summarized in Figure 3.3. This is based on Faerch and Kasper (1983:33) with the addition of the personal goal component.

What needs to be noted is that while CSs provides a means of coping with the problem, and can enable the person to reach his/her communicative goal (i.e. my goal is to ask for directions), this does not necessarily mean that this leads to successful communication (i.e. that the listener will understand the request and comply). In other words, CSs focus on the client rather than on the dynamics of the communication as a whole (Chapter 4).

Within this general framework, we can identify two basic types of strategies or behaviours. Abandoning the personal or communicative goals characterizes 'avoidance behaviour' and modifying the plan 'achievement behaviour' (Faerch and Kasper, 1983). Modifying the communicative goal can be perceived as representing both avoidance and achievement, depending on how we define the two terms. It is avoidance of the original communicative goal but at the same time it strives to achieve by formulating a related, albeit slightly different, goal. Perceiving behaviours as avoiding or achieving goals depends upon how much the original goal is changed and consequently how much the communicative needs of the individual become compromised. Whether such compromising actually matters in the long run depends upon whether the personal goal was achieved by some other means (e.g. working out the map by oneself and consequently getting from A to B) and upon emotional factors.

Within these broad categories of avoidance and achievement, more specific behaviours can be identified. We shall discuss here those which have been identified in the foreign language learning context and which we, and others (namely, Miller 1989), have encountered in clinical populations. They will be discussed within the following over-all framework, in which the avoidance strategies (following Faerch and Kasper, 1983) are subdivided into formal reduction strategies and functional reduction strategies and the achievement strategies into co-operative and non-co-operative strategies. These subcategories can be explicated as follows.

1. Formal reduction strategy: The actual language systems are reduced. For instance, a person might avoid all lexical items with a specific phoneme, thus reducing the phonological system.
2. Functional reduction strategy: The functional goals of the communication are reduced. For instance, the person may not talk about topics which he/she finds linguistically difficult.
3. Co-operative strategy: The problem is solved, or worked upon, on a co-operative basis with other interactants. For instance, the person with the difficulty can simply ask for assistance.
4. Non-co-operative strategy: The problem is solved, worked upon, by the individual alone.

The specific CSs classified within this framework are summarized in Table 3.1. This table is designed to be largely self-explanatory. Those familiar with communicative handicaps can readily identify behaviours they have encountered and which can be described in terms of these CSs. There are likely to be many others. Studies examining CSs in various clinical populations remain to be carried out.

The concept of communication strategy has much to offer for the speech-language professional. We shall consider only some more general clinical implications here. Firstly, the types of strategies used can tell us about the client's approach to life in general and to his/her handicap in particular. Trying to achieve can be a risky enterprise in that the client is exposing the disability. Employing avoidance

Table 3.1 Overview of Communication Strategies

Avoidance strategies:
I. FORMAL REDUCTION
1. Phonological
   e.g. avoids lexical items containing certain phonemes which one finds difficult to produce
2. Morphological
   e.g. avoids plurals, if have a lisp
3. Syntactic
   e.g. produces only short sentences because of problems with producing long utterances
4. Lexical
   e.g. uses only certain lexical items because not confident about the meanings of many others
II. FUNCTIONAL REDUCTION
1. Actional Reduction
   e.g. avoids certain actions and situations altogether (after a stroke stops going to the pub) or abandons exchange
2. Modal Reduction
   e.g. doesn't use all available channels of communication (because of a stutter avoids telephones)
3. Reduction of the Propositional Content
   a. topic avoidance
   e.g. doesn't talk about linguistically or otherwise difficult topics; or acts as if understands/bluffs
   b. message abandonment
   e.g. cut communication on a topic short
   c. meaning replacement
   e.g. uses a general expression when not sure what an available specific expression means exactly ('bird' for a pheasant).

Table 3.1 continued

Achievement strategies:
I. CO-OPERATIVE
1. Appeal for Assistance
   e.g. by verbal or non-verbal means asks the interlocuter to help
II. NON-CO-OPERATIVE
1. Code-switching
   e.g. switching between different styles when cannot find an appropriate expression; or bi(multi)linguals switch between different languages
2. Generalization
   e.g. uses a general expression when cannot retrieve or does not have a specific expression available ('bird' for a duck)
3. Paraphrase
   e.g. describes characteristics of an object when specific expression not available
4. Word Coinage
   e.g. create a new word for an unavailable one (neologisms)
5. Restructuring
   e.g. restructure plan which cannot be completed (such as false starts; dysfluency)
6. Non-linguistic Strategies
   e.g. mime, gesture, sound imitation

strategies can be a much safer option for those who feel unable to face their shortcomings, who feel too discouraged to continue trying to overcome their problems or who are naturally timid. Another appropriate, and at times rather descriptive term for avoidance strategies could be concealment strategies. The client is trying to hide the problems for whatever reasons. On the other hand, the use of a limited range of strategies may simply reflect the only strategies available for the client. Or, they may reflect the client's choice of opting out.

Secondly, viewing communication problems in terms of CSs is a positive approach to disability. The focus is on the underlying motivations for unusual communicative behaviours. Customarily, deviations from the norm are viewed as aspects of one's behaviour to be eradicated at any cost. This reflects a focus on form of expression rather than communicative effectiveness and functionality. Exploring clients' communicative shortcomings in terms of achievement strategies shifts the focus to communicative ability:

how could the client communicate despite the existing problems? Similarly, exploring avoidance strategies is a positive approach to disability: what is the client doing to conceal his/her disability and to what extent does this concealment compromise the client's communicative functioning? If they compromise the client's personal needs and/or hinder communication, then they may provide suitable targets for remediation. If, on the other hand, the strategies build the client's confidence by 'normalizing' communicative behaviour then they may constitute behaviours to be encouraged. As such, strategies which may involve production of linguistically 'incorrect' utterances may be encouraged for functional ends. Encouragment of achievement behaviours in particular and validation of avoidance behaviours when the client feels he or she needs them may provide appropriate therapy for those who have limited access to formal linguistic structures (Chapter 7; also Miller, 1989).

Finally, CSs can reflect the nature of the relationship between interactants. Feeling comfortable and safe in a relationship is likely to encourage one to try achievement strategies rather than playing safe by avoiding communication. Not feeling foolish or a failure and feeling that one is making some real things happen as a result of trying to communicate are conducive to achievement. Creating such safe environments may be encouraged in clinical encounters. This may involve the therapist imposing less control on the interaction, exploring the client's interests and topics with genuine interest and trying to create 'real' interactions which motivate the client to experiment further (Chapter 7).

SUMMARY

In this chapter we have discussed aspects of discourse structure and communication which we feel bear relevance for the clinical management of communication disorders. The discussion has necessarily been broad and lacking in linguistic detail; we have striven for conciseness and clarity rather than for exhaustive accounts of the phenomena. Understanding how descriptions of communicative behaviours can have different focus and motivations promotes understanding of how different descriptions can reveal different information about one's communicative ability or disability. What has been discussed in this chapter feeds directly into discussions on assessment, diagnosis and treatment of communication problems (Chapters 5, 6 and 7). Before examining these aspects of the clinical management of communication problems, we shall consider some issues in 'clinical pragmatics'.

Chapter 4

Issues in clinical pragmatics

In Chapter 2 we discussed what the study of clinical pragmatics might entail. Within a clinical pragmatic framework we are interested in

1. How positive and negative aspects of one's communicative behaviour become identified;
2. How such behaviours are described;
3. What the possible motivations and causes for the behaviours are; and
4. How pragmatic methods and principles serve clinical needs.

Considering communication within such perspective one concentrates on the process by which meanings are created rather than the actual behavioural product. Focus is on the dynamics of the communication, on the sharing of responsibility for both successful and unsuccessful interaction between the participants rather than placing it mainly on the client.

Observers tend to see what they are accustomed or trained to see. Speech-language professionals tend to rely heavily on existing analytical frameworks, drawing their attention to specific aspects of the client's communicative behaviour. While this is obviously a workable approach, guiding one's observations and enabling one to categorize them into meaningful units, there is the danger that one might fail to observe other meanings equally central to the understanding of the client as a communicator. By its very nature, an analytical framework cannot be fully comprehensive and exhaustive. Not all meaningful behaviours can be captured within one model (or any model). Not that there is any urgent need for this, since many gaps in analytical frameworks can be filled in by experienced clinicians. Yet, there are certain aspects of existing frameworks which need to be reconsidered and which we aim to highlight in this chapter and explore further in the chapter on assessment (Chapter 6).

What we propose to discuss here are some issues in clinical pragmatics, attempting to bring together those aspects of communication which we feel are particularly clinically pertinent and which can become easily undermined in analytical frameworks. More specifically, the following key questions will be explored:

1. How communicative behaviours become identified and categorized as positive/appropriate or negative/inappropriate;
2. How communicative behaviours are described;
3. How communicative behaviours come into being.

IDENTIFICATION OF COMMUNICATIVE BEHAVIOURS

Clients come to the attention of communication specialists because somebody has identified that a potential problem might exist. One can gain valuable insight into the nature of the problem and its consequent management if one tries to find out both why others find it difficult to communicate with the client, and in what circumstances others find communication enjoyable and rewarding with the client. As is suggested in Chapter 7 (see also Chapter 6), this can take the form of rather simple introspection of the form 'I find it difficult to communicate with X because . . .

1. He/she makes me feel uncomfortable.
2. I cannot follow what he/she says.
3. We don't share many common interests etc.'

And, 'I find it enjoyable to communicate with X because . . .

1. He/she makes me feel special.
2. We respect one another.
3. He/she gives me encouraging eye contact etc.'

Part of such introspection is the realization that successful and unsuccessful communication is created by all the participants and that the client's behaviour as well as our discomfort may stem from the communicative context rather than the client alone (Example 2, below). Being able to attribute some of the responsibility to oneself as a 'normally functioning' communicator or to the communicative context requires honest and searching appraisal of oneself and awareness of how meanings come into being in communication. Part of the clinical management of communication disorders is the raising of communicative awareness in those who interact with the client. Using the concepts and methods of the pragmatic approach, it is possible to devise questionnaires which explore how clients and others view one anothers' communicative strengths and weaknesses (Chapter 6). This enables one to explore the communicative responsibilities of participants and their potential roles in creating the communicative encounters, thus enabling one to evaluate the communicative abilities of the client within a communicative context. The ensuing remedial plans can build upon this, and other relevant knowledge to target problems which are real for the client as a communicator (Chapter 7).

Realization, both on the part of the client and those who interact with him or her, that a communication problem exists can take a variety of forms ranging from a clear inability to share meanings to feelings of unease. More specifically, a communication problem may surface because:

1. (One of) the participants (is) are unwilling to interact;
2. (One of) the participants cannot recover the intended meaning of an utterance;
3. (One of) the participants cannot recover the intended meaning of a non-verbal meaning expression;
4. (One of) the participants interpret(s) meanings which were expressed but not intended or read(s) more into the expression than was intended;
5. (One of) the participants find(s) the meanings expressed inappropriate;
6. (One of) the participants find(s) the other's turn-taking skills inappropriate;

7. (One of) the participants find(s) the client's communicative behaviour uncomfortable.

Exploration of matters such as these, in addition to exploration of positive aspects of interactions, in some detail could constitute a framework for the above mentioned questionnaires.

(1)–(7) can be viewed as characterizing the realization on the part of the listener that the communicative encounter is not (totally) successful or satisfying. In the clinical context, the listener, the person identifying a problem, is likely to be a partner, parent, teacher, friend of the client or a speech-language professional. The client may also recognize that a problem exists and even what the cause of the problem may be, and yet because of the communication problem may not be able to do much about it. When a client is clearly aware of the problems it is useful to try to tap into this awareness in order to gain insight and jointly plan realistic treatment programmes (Chapter 7). Yet, the client may not be able to provide a sufficiently detailed description of the problematic experiences, beyond a broad explanation of what usually goes wrong when they engage in communication (e.g. 'By the time I've thought of something to say, it's too late'; 'I always seem to say the wrong thing'; 'I don't think that people like me'). Thus, it is the task of those interacting with the client to identify and describe the problematic communicative behaviours (or to assist the client in doing so, Chapter 7). Even though the emphasis is on the client, it is important to recognize that those interacting with the client contribute towards the communicative encounter: Their behaviour, or mere existence, may facilitate or hinder communication.

(1)–(7) can be further classified according to the severity of the communication problem as perceived by the listener. Severity of a problem as reflected in the extent of disturbance to communication can be examined by considering the extent of potential disturbance to the sharing and interpretation of meanings. Thus, we can arrive at the following potential rank order:

$$\{(1) > (2) > (3)\} > (4) < (5) > (6) (7)$$

Meanings cannot be shared at all if one of the interactants is unwilling to communicate, and thus (1) is given the highest rank in relation to the others. Being unable to recover an intended meaning of an utterance, i.e. (2), is considered more detrimental than being unable to recover the intended meaning of a non-verbal meaning expression, i.e. (3), since verbal communication is the main means of communicating in most human interactive encounters. This order may however need to be qualified for those whose main means of communication are non-verbal. (4) can be considered less detrimental than the first three in that meanings are interpreted, however not the intended ones. In case of (4), the interpreted meanings are appropriate to the communicative context, while for (5) they are inappropriate and thus (5) can be considered more detrimental than (4). (6) and (7) describe communicative behaviours which do not directly affect the recoverability of meanings, and thus are considered less detrimental to signalling of meanings than all the others.

The severity rating suggests that expressing meanings inappropriately, having problems in taking turns and exhibiting behaviours which the listener finds uncomfortable are less central for communication than expression of meanings. This is true in so far that these behaviours do not arise unless one attempts to express meanings. Yet, in complex human relationships, using an impolite expression instead of a polite one, monopolizing or avoiding the floor, staring at the listener or standing too close to him/her are powerful communicative devices which signal their own meanings and which are likely to create an unfavourable impression in the mind of the listener. Indeed, people will not seek the company of those who make them feel uncomfortable. It is perhaps necessary to re-evaluate the centrality of verbal meaning expressions in communication and to consider the implications of such re-evaluation to the management of communication problems.

A communication problem may result from a clear inability to interpret meanings. There can be instances where no listener could place an interpretation onto a meaning expression and there are those expressions which can be interpreted by some but not everyone. Interpretation is not an all-or-nothing affair but hinges upon the notion of continuum. At one end of the continuum all members of the same speech community can interpret a particular expression while at the opposite end nobody can. In between these extremes are the instances where interpretation is dependent on the individual interpreters and on the various communicative contexts. For instance, the language of apparently unintelligible speakers can often be understood by those who are familiar with the speaker (e.g. Connolly, 1984). Also, contextual clues aid interpretation. When a person says [izu] and points to a pair of scissors on the table with the accompanying movement signalling 'give to me' the listener can interpret the utterance and act accordingly, if he/she so wishes.

APPROPRIATENESS VS. INAPPROPRIATENESS

In those communicative encounters where meanings are recovered and interpreted but are judged somehow unsuitable, we are concerned with the distinction of appropriate/ acceptable vs. inappropriate/unacceptable. As with any interpretation of meaning, in between the two extremes of appropriate or inappropriate to all is a grey area which is motivated by specific norms generated by sub-cultures, individual preferences, different situations, environments and relationships. While such 'norms' as 'One should not talk like that to one's parents', 'One should not interrupt without apologizing', 'One should not swear in the company of women' can be widely held within communities, any norm is ultimately specific to individuals. Individuals may choose not to conform to the general principles of appropriacy and/or can interpret the widely held views idiosyncratically. Yet, 'not anything goes' and those who deviate grossly and visibly from the general norms are often categorized as odd and difficult to communicate with (Bishop and Adams, 1989; also Chapter 6). Part of one's communicative and pragmatic competences (Chapter 5) is the ability to judge behaviours as appropriate and inappropriate within the confines of the norms of one's culture and to communicate oneself within these norms. Part of these competences is also the knowledge that one has the choice

of behaving inappropriately and that such behaviours are
likely to have certain consequences on one's life for which
one is responsible.

Another aspect of the notion of appropriacy which those
in the position of modifying others' behaviour need to be
aware of concerns people's attitudes towards 'negative'
behaviours. 'Negative' behaviours such as refusing to communicate or using abusive language are not necessarily
inappropriate. It is part of human existence to express both
positive and negative emotions and to take the resulting
consequences. Whether such expressions are judged as
appropriate or inappropriate depends on the context in
which they occur. In the clinical context, it is beneficial
in the first instance not to deem 'negative' behaviours as
inappropriate behaviours which need to be eradicated but
to explore their underlying motivations. Negative behaviours serve as a window to one's inner problems, be they
pragmatic, emotional or whatever in nature. Also, behaving always appropriately can in itself be an indication of
an underlying problem: 'I cannot cope with others being
upset with me' or 'I don't know how to express negative
feelings'. One should not forget either that everyone has the
right to choose to behave 'inappropriately' and to signal the
associated negative meanings. One may choose to leave a
room without saying anything, wanting to signal some such
meanings as 'I don't care how you feel' or 'I want to make
you feel upset'. Or, there is always the possibility that
one is behaving inappropriately simply because one is pre-
occupied or distracted, and thus not aware of what one is
doing. In all these instances, a person can be said to be
behaving 'appropriately inappropriately' and whether one
considers such behaviours as problematic depends on how
those coming across such behaviours can deal with negative
behaviour (i.e. whether they feel threatened by it).

In addition to decisions concerning the appropriacy of
communicative occurrences, listeners can also judge behaviours as problematic if they are difficult to process. In
other words, if the listener has to work hard (inference
hard) to place an interpretation onto a meaning expression,
it can be judged communicatively inefficient (de Beaugrande
and Dressler, 1981). In the context of a joke or literature,

this might obviously be considered subtle or powerful. In the clinical context, it is important to know whether an expression is difficult to process because of something the client does or fails to do or because of the influences bearing upon the interpretation by others.

DESCRIPTION OF COMMUNICATIVE BEHAVIOURS: EXPLORATION OF HOW THE BEHAVIOURS COME INTO BEING

Having identified that a communication problem exists, presumably on the basis of some such general guidelines as outlined above, the task is then to describe the communicative phenomena. We can distinguish between informal description and description within an analytical framework. The latter is more focused and systematic, both of which have positive and negative implications. Systematic description is a way of organizing one's initial observations into a more detailed and informative format, which then helps to clarify the nature of the problem and enables one to speculate on its possible causes (see below). But, working within a framework can restrict one's observations only to the categories which form part of the framework and thus one might fail to observe other aspects of behaviour which are also important. Systematic description is a means of categorizing and labelling behaviour. It is a powerful device which directs and focuses one's attention to particular aspects of behaviour rather than others. Given that no framework can be fully exhaustive, one needs to be aware of how to assess the strengths and weaknesses of analytical tools and one must not assume that if a procedure claims to assess the 'whole of one's communicative competence' it ever manages to do so (Chapter 6).

Descriptive frameworks of communicative phenomena occurring in the clinical context need to be motivated by the clinical aims of clarifying problems and devising remedial measures. Labelling and describing are likely to be less useful when not done for a specific purpose. The aim of analysing communication within the clinical pragmatic framework is to arrive at descriptions which shed light on the client's ability or inability to share meanings with others and which consequently lead to valuable and realistic treatment programmes. It serves no purpose to observe that a client does not do something without considering why and without considering what effect this has on him/her and others. A clinical pragmatic framework aims to identify and describe those behaviours which matter to the client as a communicator and consequently work on this basis. In other words, one does not focus on aspects of communication simply because they are part of communication, or part of an analytical tool, but rather on those which have value and reality for the client. To take a concrete example, one would not work on a phonological system if the client did not have concepts in the first place. As one of our colleagues put it, clinicians at times work 'on the tread of the tyres when the engine is at fault'.

There are certain basic features which tools for describing communicative behaviours need to possess for being maximally valuable in the clinical context. These are features which are motivated by the clinical aims of diagnosis and remediation.

1. Focus on the basic features of communication without which communication would be very difficult, if not impossible.
2. Focus on aspects of communication, specific to cultures and contexts.
3. Focus not only on those aspects of communication which can be accurately described but also on one's hunches and feelings which cannot be explored in precise terms.
4. Focus not only on the client's behaviour but on the behaviour of all the interactants and consider their roles in creating the communicative event.
5. Focus on other contextual influences on the communicative event.
6. Focus not only on problematic behaviours but also on successful ones.
7. Make judgements about the communicative value of behaviours and consider motivations for the judgements.
8. Make judgements of whether particular behaviours are appropriate or inappropriate and consider why.
9. Make judgements about the facilitative and non-

facilitative nature of behaviours and consider why they operate in this way.
10. Focus on one's own assumptions and biases as an observer (Eastwood, 1988).

Let us consider each of these in more detail.

1. If the purpose of the description of communicative behaviours is to shed light on one's communicative ability and disability, it needs to begin with the very basics of communication. If, as we maintain, being able to share meanings with others is based on being able to 'communicate' within oneself, the first aim of description would be to explore the ability of all the interactants to do this (Chapter 1). This can take the form of exploring the participants' interests, their concepts, thoughts and feelings and the way these are connected. It is also valuable to give some attention to those thoughts and feelings which are not expressed ('I wonder why this person never mentions their disability'). This kind of exploration can enhance one's understanding of what communication involves. It also highlights the fact that topics can be shared or unshared and that ideas may or may not be valid and interesting for exterior communication. Choosing not to comment on something unappealing in order not to hurt another person's feelings involves making the distinction between interior and exterior validity. Most people know someone who is not very skilled at this. More extreme examples occur with neurological damage where the necessary ability to inhibit may not be present (Perecman, 1987, Code, 1989). Everyone interested in communication has a legitimate interest in interior communication. It is not just the domain of psychologists, counsellors, psychotherapists, psychiatrists and poets, neither is it something which need only be addressed when an emotional problem arises.

When focusing on exterior communication, the first step would be to identify whether a person interacts with others at all, and if so with whom and to what effect (Gallagher, 1983, Chapter 6). Finding out from clients and their communicative partners the contexts in which communication is successful or unsuccessful and why is part of clinical appraisal. When focusing on specific behaviours one would

include descriptions of the basic interactional structures of
initiation and response, of opening-, middle- and closing-
sequences and of turn-taking dynamics (Chapter 3). These
descriptions would capture the basic structures of interactional communication which is based on a person expressing something and another person somehow re-acting to
this expression.

2. Within this overall structure finer descriptive categories
can then be identified. These would include explorations
into what the interactants try to achieve with their meaning
expressions and whether they do so (intentionality, Chapter
1, speech acts, Chapter 3), how ideas and topics are developed individually and through negotiation (coherence,
Chapter 3), how expressions are linked to form larger structures (cohesion, Chapter 3) and how much information
utterances carry (informativity, Chapter 3). One would also
be interested in examining how communication problems
are dealt with. This involves examination of repair and
clarification behaviours and of strategies which are devised
to overcome communication problems (communication
strategies, Chapter 3). When examinining any of the communicative behaviours one would describe both verbal and
non-verbal expressions of meaning.

In addition to describing the above kinds of pragmatic
and discourse phenomena, description of communicative phenomena includes linguistic analysis of the client's
language, examination of general cognitive and motor skills
and evaluation of how they relate to the client's ability or
inability to communicate. These types of analyses and assessments need to be considered as part of the wider framework of communicative assessment. This link needs to be
emphasized particularly in relation to clinical linguistic
analyses which at times tend to consider linguistic systems as
somewhat separate from communication. This point will be
discussed further in Example 3, below. Appraisal of the
linguistic, cognitive, motor and perceptual skills constitutes a
means of exploring the possible causes of communicative
problems.

3. As is apparent from Chapter 3, descriptive frameworks
exist for examining the above kinds of communicative
phenomena. One should not however restrict one's obser-

vation and description to include only those behaviours which fit neatly within the existing descriptive categories. Keeping track of one's hunches and intuitions about what is happening in specific communicative encounters is an integral part of clinical observation. Identification of what descriptive frameworks fail to capture is as essential as identifying the behaviours they address. It is also essential to appreciate that clients, and all interactants, have the right not to engage in communication if they so wish and that gaps in behaviour resulting from such motivations need also to be identified and described in a clinical approach. Recently, a client of ours who had been unable to follow narratives prior to therapy exercised his right to look quietly at every picture in a story book. This took some time but was allowed by the therapist, who was rewarded by a subsequent satisfactory discussion of the story (see also Tough, 1973).

4. While the client is understandably the focus of attention in the clinical context, one is also interested in describing some of the communicative behaviours of those interacting with the client. This enables one to examine how the client's communicative behaviours may have come into being as a result of the behaviours of others (see Example 1, below). For instance, it is well-documented that specific types of initiation produce specific types of response. Thus, if a client produced minor utterances such as 'yes', 'no' and 'don't know' we would be able to examine whether these reflected the client's communicative ability or closed questions requiring such responses (e.g. Crystal, Fletcher and Garman, 1976, Tough, 1976). Which behaviours of the others one would focus upon depends on what the clinician perceives as having a potential effect on the client's behaviour. There are no all-embracing guidelines.

5. Focusing on the potential influences which may create the communicative behaviours of the client and others, one would also wish to consider such contextual factors as the physical context in which the event takes place, the type of task, activity or interaction one is engaged in and the personal and professional relationships existing between the interactants. The question one wishes to ask is how such influences can affect, positively and negatively, the

behaviours of the individuals. It is, for instance, particularly helpful to know for remediation whether certain activities or clinician-client relationships are conducive to the (re)learning of skill (Chapter 7). A more general exploration of with whom, in what contexts and to what effect the client communicates is also an important aspect of clinical appraisal (Gallagher, 1983).

Part of one's examination of the contextual influences is an exploration of the metacommunicative behaviours taking place in interactions (Chapter 3). Who organizes and directs the communicative flow can be indicative of who has the most influence on the communicative behaviours of others. One would assume that in equal encounters, in which the communicative load is fairly evenly shared, the influences upon one another are also fairly even. In clinical encounters in particular we are concerned with those influences which can be said to have some negative effects. What exactly these negative effects would be is largely dependent on the individuals concerned. For instance, one person may cease to communicate if being explicitly criticized while another person may try to change the behaviours concerned (Chapter 3). Observing the kinds of metacommunications taking place in interactions and trying to evaluate their (potential) effects is a way of describing communication with a view to understanding why the client may behave in certain ways in certain situations.

6. Even though one is ultimately interested in finding out whether a communication problem exists and what the nature of it is, one is also interested in exploring how and when the client communicates successfully. Determining what constitutes successful communication would need to be modified according to the specific disabilities of clients. Exploring strengths as well as weaknesses provides a basis upon which realistic treatment programmes can be built (Chapter 7).

7. and 8. Part of the consideration of what the client is capable of doing is the appraisal of the communicative value of behaviours. All behaviours communicate something, albeit only that one is not able to communicate or wishes not to do so. Thus, there is no decision as to whether behaviours are communicative or not. What one can focus

upon, however, is whether the behaviours communicate what the person intended. Thus, exploring whether a client is able to communicate involves exploration of what the client is aiming to achieve with the specific behaviours and whether these goals are achieved. It also involves exploration of unintentionally communicated meanings and meanings which the listeners read into expressions (Chapter 1, intentionality). As such, a simple division of communicative vs. non-communicative does not exist but rather we are concerned with the notion of intentionality and its role in creating successful and unsuccessful communication.

Investigation of the communicative value of behaviours also involves judgements about the appropriacy and inappropriacy of behaviours. These issues were discussed in the above section on 'Identification of communicative behaviours' as these notions can be envisaged as characterizing one's initial feelings of communication being 'normal' or somehow 'disordered'. Recording whether communicative behaviours are judged as appropriate or inappropriate, and why, can be considered part of analytical frameworks (Chapter 6).

9. In the clinical context, part of such a framework is also an assessment of the 'therapeutic' value of the behaviours of those interacting with the client. This can take the form of deciding whether the behaviours of others can be considered facilitative, non-facilitative or neither and why. These are very crude distinctions which can be refined incorporating contextual information into the decision-making process. For instance, a warning frown can be facilitative to a skilled and confident performer but non-facilitative to a nervous beginner. Making such statements about the communicative behaviours of others involves informed and honest appraisal of the behaviours of all the interactants, including evaluation of the clinical management methods of the clinicians themselves. Again, it can take the form of a directed self-exploration of how the interactants see their behaviour aiding or hindering the communicative process, and specifically affecting the client's behaviour. It is also essential to explore how the client perceives the role of others. Since it is often very difficult to evaluate one's own behaviour, and in particular to identify problems with it, it may also

be necessary to seek the opinion of an 'unbiased', but informed, observer. At a practical level, one can envisage questionnaires guiding one's observations and judgements which can then be compared for the various individuals concerned with the communicative event (or the client).

10. Recognizing that observation and description can be coloured by the assumptions, biases and prejudices of the observer renders description potentially valid. An extreme example would be assuming that all people who shout are domineering and therefore missing the fact that one of the interactants is hard of hearing.

CONCLUSIONS

As is apparent from the above, description of communicative behaviours is motivated by wanting to know how the actual behaviours of a client come into existence. Clinical observation does not simply consist of the labelling of behaviours but also consideration of their communicative consequences and of their possible causes. As such, description and labelling are motivated by evaluation and explanation. Similarly, the exploration of the causes of behaviours is motivated by description. Descriptive categories focus one's attention on particular causes and influences. It is thus essential to consider the two together in the clinical appraisal of communicative ability in order not to consider description as an end in itself. It is our belief that categorization and labelling of clients' behaviours are not always fully thought out. Questions such as 'What does it really mean when a client uses deictic items inappropriately?', 'Why isn't the client initiating?' or 'Why is the client interrupting unnecessarily?' are sometimes left unasked. It is known to us that clients can become diagnosed as pragmatically disordered solely on the basis of their problems being describable in terms of pragmatic categories such as initiation-response, speech acts or discourse structures (Chapter 6). Similarly, consider a client who is diagnosed as grammatically disordered because he/she tends to delete grammatical subjects in certain contexts. This observation and consequent diagnosis can be misleading unless we consider why subjects are variably deleted. It may be that the client is deleting the grammatical subject when the deleted information can be recovered by the listener (i.e. 'known', Chapter 3) but does not do so when the information is unknown. What in the surface structure can appear as a grammatical problem may in fact reflect the client's means of dealing with an underlying cognitive problem of handling longer sequences of language. Or the client may not have a problem but may simply regard structure as a vehicle of communication rather than an end in itself. Labelling someone disordered is rather meaningless unless we try to explore fully why and how the specific behaviours come into being (Chapter 6). We believe that an explanatory component is not an aspect of the clinical process which can be given some thought after observation and description have been completed. It is an integral part of the descriptive process because describing with a view to explaining influences the nature of the description.

What has been considered here under the heading of 'clinical pragmatics' is in no way a novel idea. It brings together ideas from social skills training, from speech therapy, counselling and psychotherapy. What we hope to do by bringing many of these rather diverse approaches into the context of communicative disability is to highlight that speech-language professionals, communication specialists, need to consider that the client's handicap is likely to emerge as a consequence of the interaction of many factors both inside and outside the client. This is not to claim that this has not indeed been the focus of much of the clinical literature in recent years, particularly in the USA, but to maintain that it is useful to discuss the rather fragmented approaches to pragmatics in the clinical context within one model or framework. One can easily lose the appreciation that the various component parts of communication, which often, and necessarily, form the basis for clinical study are indeed components of a bigger whole and in order to be fully meaningful and functioning need at some point to be considered within the context of that whole.

What has been discussed here forms rather an idealistic view of clinical practice. Exploring the various factors which shape communication and influence communicative dis-

ability is a time-consuming process. The training of clinicians, at least in the UK, and the time allowed for retrain-
ing and further development of knowledge and skill while
working may not be sufficient for adequate mental preparation and acquisition of knowledge which are required
for honest and exhaustive appraisal of the dynamics of
clinical communicative encounters and the client's communicative ability. Working within the kind of model described here would be a process which would not take
place in one or two clinical sessions but over a longer period
of time. It is also a tool which does not lend itself to norm-
related scores but rather enables one to delve into the deeper
meanings in interaction and therapy. It is also a clinical
framework which places emphasis on observation, description and exploration before actual remediation and thus
one which may seem threatening to clinicians whose professional obligations may encourage 'doing therapy' rather
than engaging in activities which may not appear in the
early stages as treating the client at all (Chapter 7). Some of
the guidelines suggested here can also be threatening to
those whose behaviour is being analysed. Clinicians would
need to take great care not to make any of the interactants
feel negative towards the possibility of having to change
behaviour which is not facilitative or appropriate. In practice this is not likely to be easy. Similarly, clinicians need
not to feel professionally undermined if it surfaces that in
fact their own behaviour can be somehow restricting. It is a
healthy attitude towards oneself and one's work to accept
that nobody is, or needs to be, perfect.

We shall now consider three examples which highlight
the issues discussed. In Example 1, we shall consider how
our perception of children's ability to repair and clarify can
be affected by contextual factors. We shall discuss certain aspects of a case study of Christopher which we have
explored elsewhere in more detail (Leinonen and Smith,
1989). In Example 2, we shall focus on the level of discourse
structure, and consider how analysis of incohesion in discourse can be motivated and guided by the principles of
clinical pragmatics. In Example 3, issues involved in considering linguistic levels as interacting entities, serving a
communicative function, are briefly discussed.

Example 1   129

EXAMPLE 1 CONTEXTUAL INFLUENCES ON CHILDREN'S
REPAIR AND CLARIFICATION

It is often on the basis of observable behaviours of clients
that we make inferences about the clients' ability or inability to communicate. Focusing on children's initiations
of and responses to clarifications and repairs, these behaviours can tell us a great deal about a child as a communicator. These behaviours can be indicative of children's
developing skills as co-operative partners in communication, of their ability to attend to and understand the messages of others, their ability to monitor their own comprehension and to appreciate the deficiences of their own
messages (Fey, Warr-Leeper, Webber and Disher, 1988).
They also reflect children's awareness of the social obligation to repair and their assertiveness and perception of self-
worth. A great many conclusions about communicative
ability can be drawn by simply observing clarification and
repair behaviours in communication. It is thus important
to appreciate that the child's behaviours do not necessarily
stem from the child but can surface from the dynamics of
the communication. In order to avoid misassessment and
misdiagnosis, it is thus essential to work within a clinical
pragmatic approach.

When considering repair and clarification (or any communicative phenomenon) in the clinical context, it does not
suffice simply to record whether these behaviours occur or
do not occur (e.g. McTear, 1985a) but one also needs to
consider motivating factors. We shall focus on instances
where misassessment and misdiagnosis may result from
analysis and observation not taking into account the following issues:

1. From what perspective are we assessing the behaviours?
2. Are those interacting with children interpreting behaviours within predetermined discourse plans?
3. What are the underlying motivations and responsibilities
   of all the interactants in communication and how can
   they shape the interaction?
4. Are the clarifications and repairs successful?
5. What effect can different types of clarification and repair
   stimuli have on responses?

6. What are the 'real' functions of repair and clarification requests?

Failing to consider such questions when assessing children's ability to clarify and repair can obscure our view of children's ability to communicate successfully. Let us consider each of the seven points in more detail to explore how one's judgements can be obscured.

1. People studying children's communication are essentially adults and consequently behaviours are perceived and evaluated from an adult's perspective. There can be instances where behaviours which are perfectly natural to children are judged inappropriate on the basis of an adult frame of reference. Leinonen and Smith (1989) consider the following example to illustrate this point. Imagine that two men are conversing over their beer. One has been asked which race he intends to be in at the forthcoming village sports day. He replies that, ideally, he would like to be in X (a town several miles from the village). His companion is likely to laugh and understand that village sports are amongst the friend's least favourite activities. However, a speech therapist conversing with a ten year old pupil in McTear (1985a, 246–247) continues the conversation very differently.

Sp.Th. Which race would you like to be in?
Child. I like to be in X (a town several miles from the school) in the sports day.
Sp.Th. In X?
Child. Yes
Sp.Th. What do you mean?
Child. I mean something.
Sp.Th. Is there a sports day in X?
Child. There is not there is a sports day in Y (the school).
Sp.Th. Then what's X got to do with it?
Child. Nothing.
Sp.Th. Then why did you mention it?
Child. Indeed I did mention it.
Sp.Th. Why did you mention it?
Child. I don't know.

While this conversation clearly indicates the child's failure to provide the information sought by the adult, from the

Example 1 131

child's point of view an attempt might have been made to say what one as a child is often forbidden to say: 'I hate sports days and would rather be anywhere else than at one'. It is interesting to compare the response of the adult to the child's utterances with the hypothetical, but in our view realistic, exchange between two adults discussing the same topic. Quite clearly adults impose different conversational rules and rights when interacting with children than when interacting with adults. Amongst adults, equal conversational rights are more likely to prevail. In this example, the adult assumes the right to demand a satisfactory answer, which is reflected in the two instances of 'Why did you mention it?' This example can also be seen as reflecting the adult's view of what children should like and not like. The adult seems to operate with the assumption that 'Children ought to enjoy sports days and ought to say so' and everything said by the child is interpreted and evaluated within this frame. This approach differs from one which simply feeds back to the child the fact that he/she has not been understood.

Considering that children's conversational rights may be unrealistically suspended by adults and that children's behaviours are often evaluated within predetermined frames of interpretation based on adult reality are crucial in the clinical context. Assuming on the basis of the above example, for instance, that the child cannot repair and clarify could be a gross misjudgement of ability. While clinicians are clearly aware of such possible misguided diagnosis, it is not uncommon to find children's behaviours described as unsuccessful on such a false premise. Consider, for instance, the following examples from Brinton and Fujuki (1982, 60, 61). The contributions marked by (*) are considered as inappropriate responses (i.e. non-clarifications) to the clarification requests.

Two children are engaged in a free-play situation.
1. A. Oh. What is it?
    B. ⟨continues to sing a nonsense song⟩ (*)
2. A. I wonder how they get all these things?
    B. Huh?
    A. I got a basket. (*)

Clearly, these are only instances of inappropriate responses, indicative of one's inability to clarify, if we assume that all clarification requests in all interactions normally become clarified, which is untrue. In other words, we suspend children's conversational rights to play according to their own rules and have their own motivations for interactions which can, and do, differ from those of adults. Considering children's communicative behaviours from children's perspective is often difficult, and appears particularly difficult in clinical and pedagogic encounters, reflecting the motivation to correct and manage children's behaviour. Correction and management may well be appropriate in some circumstances. What, however, needs to be borne in mind is that when adults suspend certain rights in such situations, children might not realize that this has occurred and thus might not perform as expected. One needs to be aware how clinical interaction might compromise the communicative rights of children, whether such compromises are essential for the learning of skills, whether children themselves are aware that this has occurred and how such compromising might affect children's behaviours, and potentially the clinician's view of the child's ability to communicate. Similar questions need to be asked when interacting with communicatively handicapped individuals of any age. Communicative rights become easily suspended by those who are in the 'stronger' position of being 'normally functioning'.

2. The notion that adults' view of children's communicative success or failure can become obscured because of predetermined frames of interpretation (Levinson, 1983) is also relevant in the clinical context. As in the McTear example, one may fail to observe many meanings if one is operating with a fixed frame of reference. Leinonen and Smith (1989) observed interaction between a speech therapist and an eight-year-old communicatively handicapped boy, C, and concluded that because of the dynamics of such pedagogic interaction, at times an impression of successful and smooth communication was created (Chapter 3). By successful and smooth one means interaction where only few if any repair and clarification attempts surface. It appeared that this type of impression emerged because the therapist was operating within a predetermined frame of

Example 1 133

action and interpretation in which the therapist controls the topic and only asks questions for which C knows the answer (cf. Sinclair and Coulthard, 1975). Also, the only topics initiated by C which are elaborated upon are those which are about the predetermined discourse topic. Uninterpretable utterances not critical to the plan tend also not to become clarified. The following is an extract from a conversation between C and his therapist.

T. What colour is a sunflower?
C. Black leaves.
  And a bit of black in the middle.
T. Yes, but what colour are the petals?
C. Green.
T. No.
  The leaves are green.
  What colour is the flower?
C. The leaves are yellow.
  And then there is a black bit.
  And there is a green stalk.
T. That's right.
C. And the roots grow.
  And they didn't have them green things.
T. ⟨no attempt at clarifying the above apparently uninterpretable utterance⟩
  Is it a big flower or a little flower?
C. A big giant one.
T. That's right.
  It is, isn't it?

Failing to consider the various characteristics of this pedagogic register and its potential influences on the behaviour of C could lead one to believe that C is a more able communicator than he actually is in other contexts. It is also necessary to evaluate the function of such conversations about apparently trivial topics in speech therapy. Do they promote the learning and use of skill? (Chapter 7.) One aspect of therapy based on clinical pragmatic principles is to engage in activities and converse on topics which are real and, at least to some degree, significant for the interactants (Chapter 7).
  3. The above example highlights the importance of con-

sidering the motivations and responsibilities of all the interactants in shaping the communicative event. If we consider
the 'sports day' example of McTear's (1985a), it is quite
possible that the child's inadequate powers of repair and
the therapist's 'corrective' attitude combine to create a situation in which communication breakdown is inevitable.
Similarly, in the above 'sunflower' example the child's
behaviours are quite probably constrained and shaped
by the behaviour of the therapist. It is part of a realistic
appraisal of communication breakdown to share some of
the responsibility for failure. This is not to suggest that one
as a 'normally functioning' individual would be somehow
responsible if one couldn't understand unintelligible speech
but rather to emphasize the need to consider the roles of all
participants in creating communication.

What we would also like to emphasize is that in addition
to more global motivations which shape communicative
events, they can also be affected by motivations which
change throughout the interaction. Communication events
can be envisaged as reflecting different purposes. Within
one event, which has a beginning, a middle and an end,
there can be many communicative forces and motivations
which shape the specific communicative episodes (Levinson,
1983). In their exploration of C's communicative behaviour,
Leinonen and Smith (1989) observed three distinct motivations which appeared to affect the way the communication
unfolded and consequently how one perceived and evaluated
C's ability to communicate. In addition to the 'pedagogic
mode' already discussed, there were two contrasting motivations: that of 'let's get C to chat mode' and a 'research
mode' which had an interesting effect on the communication. When the adults were operating within the 'let's get C
to chat mode' the aim was to converse informally without
too much conflict, letting C control topical development.
Consequently, C's uninterpretable utterances were not
seriously challenged: When operating within this mode the
adults almost colluded with C's communication problems.
When operating within the 'research mode' the aim of one
of the adults was to 'explore C's ability to repair' and consequently C's unprocessable utterances were seriously and
persistently challenged. Consequently C attempted to face

Example 1   135

the communicative inefficiency of his utterances by trying to clarify. The point we wish to make is that recognizing the potential effects of different motivations underlying communicative episodes enables one to examine variability in communicative behaviour, to identify facilitative and non-facilitative contexts and to evaluate communicative success more realistically.

4. Indeed it does not simply suffice to observe that certain communicative behaviours occur, it also needs to be determined how communicative the interactants find the meanings expressed. Referring to the case of C, he can be observed to answer clarification and repair requests, yet these answers tend not to clarify the message to the listener. In the following example, for instance, C confirms appropriately for him (*) but not for the listener.

C. The school is brave.
T. The school is brave?
C. Yeah. (*)
T. Oh.
   Are you brave?

It is thus not sufficient simply to record whether clarifications and repairs occur, but it is necessary to evaluate whether they achieved their communicative goal of actually clarifying the message. In doing so, one would try to interpret the meanings both from one's own and from the child's perspective.

5. In the above example it does not suffice to say that C's answer does not clarify the meaning of the utterance 'The school is brave?' but one needs also to consider possible causes for this. One possible cause is the type of stimulus acting as a request. In the above example C interpreted the clarification request as a request for confirmation and thus his answer is appropriate. This interpretation is likely to stem from C not seeing anything wrong with his initial assertion. Compare the above example with the following hypothetical one.

A. The school is very big.
B. The school is very big?
A. Yeah.

B. Oh.
I hadn't realized.

It may be difficult for C to distinguish between his imaginary world and the world that is real to others, and thus a more explicit clarification request such as 'I cannot see how a school can be brave. People can be brave, but not schools. Can you try to tell me why you said that the school is brave?' might be more facilitative. Thus, when considering how particular communicative behaviours come into being and how communication can be maximally facilitated, one might need to consider the potential effects of stimuli on expression and interpretation of meanings.

6. 'The school is brave' example also illustrates the 'Let's get C to chat mode' where the adults are not truly interested in the sharing of meaning but rather in keeping the conversation alive. One aspect of this mode is that clarification and repair requests carry many other functions than just the function of aiming to clarify messages. In any conversation, not all clarification requests serve the function of clarifying messages but can be used to acknowledge, to encourage, to teach, to fill in turns and to show surprise (Corsaro, 1977; Olsen-Fulero, 1982). It is necessary to examine what the true functions of clarification requests are in order not to draw unwarranted conclusions about one's ability or inability to clarify and repair communication breakdown. In C's case, many of the clarification requests appeared to have the function of 'turn fillers' and thus C is not really required to clarify. This in turn is a likely reflection of the contrived nature of the interaction where the sharing of meaning does not really matter. In such a context, it is then not surprising if C did not clarify successfully, even if he was capable of doing so.

EXAMPLE 2 INCOHESION IN DISCOURSE

The general principles of clinical pragmatics are also useful when exploring discourse structures in the clinical context. Cohesion, which refers to explicit signalling of the linking of ideas and the kinds of relationships holding between them, is an aspect of discourse which can tell a great deal

Example 2 137

about one's communicative ability and about the ability to share meanings with others (Chapter 3). Signalling underlying coherence in discourse explicitly by the use of cohesive items is often necessary for interpretation of discourse connections by listeners. The speaker needs to be able to determine what the listener can process, what the listener already knows and consequently what will make the linking of ideas more efficient for the listener. While cohesion is an aspect of discourse structure included in some clinical assessment programs (Prutting and Kirchener, 1983; McTear, 1985a), it appears that its meaning is not always fully explored. What seems to happen in the clinical context is that the presence and more frequently the absence of cohesive items is noted without considering how they came or failed to come into being and what consequences they have on communication. We shall outline an approach here, based on Leinonen-Davies' (1984, 1988b) work on incohesion in foreign language learner compositions, which considers motivations for incohesion in discourse.

Let us begin by considering how discourse can be incohesive. Considering first how the listener is likely to identify a problem in cohesion enables one then to explore what the client may or may not have done for the problem to surface. A problem in cohesion is likely to be identified when the listener

1. cannot link meaning expressions together at all;
2. has to work hard to establish a link. In this instance, the piece of discourse can be said to be incohesive because of being inefficient (de Beaugrande and Dressler, 1981);
3. establishes a link but one which is not plausible in the context;
4. finds the linking of utterances uncharacteristic of the text-type in question.

There is obviously something either present or absent in the actual piece of discourse to make the listener feel that it is incohesive, on the basis of some such feelings as described in 1–4. There are two main possibilities. Either a cohesive item is missing where it should have occurred or a cohesive item is present but inappropriately used. Both of these can make the listener feel any of the above. For instance, if a cohesive item is absent, a listener may not be able to establish a link at all or may be able to establish a link by processing hard, or establishes a non-viable link. To make 1 and 4 more concrete let us consider examples of surface expressions which might have such consequences.

1. C. The boy's asleep.
      The gorilla eats a banana.
      Rides a bike. (*)
   A. Who does?
   C. The gorilla.

Here (*) C's expression lacks a cohesive item (the gorilla; lexical cohesion; Chapter 3) which makes it impossible for the listener to link this utterance to the previous one which is necessary for its full interpretation (see also informativity, Chapter 3).

2. A. Had a good time at the party.
      Didn't see you there.
      Oh. He did say.
   B. Who? Oh John. Yes I told him.

Here the reference of the item 'he' is not specified and thus B has to inference fairly hard to make the appropriate connection (e.g. The party was at John's; I told him a while back that I might not be there).

3. C. In the zoo.
      The gorilla eats bananas.
      He cleans the cages. (*)
   A. What? The gorilla?
   C. No. The keeper.

Here (*) the cohesive item 'he' (deictic reference item) related inappropriately to 'the gorilla'. An interpretation is placed but an inappropriate one.

4. 'My favourite pet'
   I like dogs. Dogs are nice and furry. Dogs can bite you and dogs bark. Dogs can be taken for walks. Dogs are man's best friend.

Here the repetition of the word 'dog' to create cohesion can be considered inefficient (de Beaugrande and Dressler, 1981)

Example 2 139

and not characteristic of the text type 'story' (cf. the text type 'list'). Depending on the age and ability of this text producer, one might expect some of the occurrences to be replaced by the reference item 'they' (cf. children's writing; Kress, 1982).

By examining the listeners' reactions to incohesion in discourse we can identify instances of incohesion which are more detrimental to communication than others. Not being able to infer the intended cohesive links at all is more detrimental than when the problem reflects other types of processing difficulty. In this interpretation emphasis is placed on the exchange of meanings. There is likely to be a point at which processing difficulties can be equally disturbing to communication as the inability to share meanings. For instance, if processing becomes too challenging or unchallenging and continues to be so for some length of time, the listener is likely to switch off, and thus meanings are not shared at all.

It is also likely that the absence or inappropriate use of certain cohesive items may be more detrimental than others. While the recoverability of meanings ultimately depends on the context, it can be hypothezised that problems with reference items, substitution, ellipsis and lexical cohesion are likely to be more detrimental than problems with conjunction. This hypothesis rests upon the fact that conjunctives signal links between larger chunks of discourse, thus aiding processing rather than being crucial for processing (Chapter 3). The appropriate use of reference items, substitution, ellipsis and lexical cohesion, however, can often be more essential for processing to be possible at all. This becomes apparent if we compare the examples 1 and 3 above with the following:

> I like dogs. Dogs are nice and furry. Dogs can bite you and dogs bark (though). (I like dogs because) Dogs can be taken for walks. (On the other hand) I don't like cats.

Adding some such linking devices (conjunctives) as in the brackets indicates explicitly to the listener how the sentences link into a larger frame of interpretation. They are not however totally essential. The links can be made without them. This is not to say that there are no instances where conjunctives make all the difference to interpretation and where the inappropriate use of reference items and such does not, but to suggest that there is this general tendency which can be of clinical use when planning remediation.

Having identified on the basis of some such feelings as outlined above that the discourse is not (fully) cohesive the task of the clinician is to describe what exactly it is in the surface text that gives rise to incohesion and how the incohesion came into being. We have already discussed that in broad terms incohesion reflects absence of cohesive items or their inappropriate use, and that identification of these is dependent on the context. Context includes the processing capacity of the listener, the possibility of cohesion being created exophorically (in reference to the physical context; Chapter 3) and the possibility of repairing the incohesion in face to face interaction. In reference to the last point, one's evaluation of incohesion would vary depending on whether there was the possibility to clarify. Thus, in writing, in non-interactive spoken discourse such as television news or some form of presentation, it is more paramount to signal cohesion explicitly and unambiguously.

For one to be able to explore cohesion and incohesion in discourse meaningfully and in clinically relevant terms, and to be able to share one's views with others it does not suffice to say that a cohesive item is inappropriate or absent. What is needed is a more refined descriptive framework which is then explored further in terms of what one needs to be able to do or did not do for the piece of discourse to be cohesive. And as emphasized throughout this chapter, the descriptive framework needs to focus not only on what the client fails to do but also what the client can do successfully. Thus, a framework needs to focus on cohesion as well as incohesion.

Exploration of what cohesive categories tell us about the client's communicative ability or inability can begin with the question of what one needs to be able to do to produce cohesive discourse. And more specifically, what one needs to be able to do to link expressions appropriately via reference, substitution, ellipsis, lexical cohesion and conjunction (Halliday and Hasan, 1976; Chapter 3). For all of these types

Example 2 141

of cohesive device one needs to be able to link events in one's mind, hold information in one's memory, pay attention and have the linguistic means of signalling the relationships. For reference, substitution, ellipsis and lexical cohesion this linking is more local while for conjunction one needs to be able to hold bigger chunks of discourse in memory. For conjunction, one also needs to be able to identify the logical relationships such as 'cause-effect', 'the opposite of' or 'in addition to' which manifest between larger chunks of discourse. For all of the devices one also needs to be able to assess what the listener can process, what the listener knows and whether information can be recovered from the extralinguistic context, in order to know how explicit the signalling of cohesion needs to be. For reference, substitution and ellipsis, for instance, one needs to ascertain that the information needed for the interpretation of meanings of these cohesive items is indeed recoverable for the listener. As such, cohesion requires the general ability to presuppose (Levinson, 1983). One also needs to perceive oneself in space and time, separate from other humans and from objects.

Such considerations of what one needs to be able to do then lead to suggestions of what one might be failing to do when producing incohesive discourse. This in turn leads to suggestions for remedial goals. On the basis of such considerations one can also evaluate the descriptive categories themselves. If linking expressions via reference and substitution, for instance, are based on more or less the same abilities, do they constitute separate descriptive categories? The answer to this question hinges upon an answer to another question. Would clinical management differ for teaching a client to create cohesion in discourse via reference rather than via substitution? The answer is likely to be negative. The categories of reference and substitution, being based on the concept of one lexical item being replaced by another, are however likely to have separate status from ellipsis, lexical cohesion and conjunction which have different clinical consequences and motivations. (These issues will be pursued further in future publications.) Analytical frameworks can then be evaluated on the basis of the clinical motivations underlying the descriptive categories. It is our belief that the motivations for clinical tools may not always be fully worked out (Chapter 6).

EXAMPLE 3 INTERACTION OF LINGUISTIC LEVELS

Being concerned with communicative ability and disability as holistic phenomena, clinical pragmatics also examines the value of separating linguistic levels in the study of communication pathology. Speech-language professionals frequently deal with language impairments which are considered specific in regard to the level of language which is being primarily affected. Hence the terms articulatory (phonetic), phonological, grammatical and discourse/pragmatic disorder or delay (for a discussion concerning the number of analytical levels in linguistic analysis, see e.g. Crystal, 1981, 1987). As theoretical constructs such specific language impairments do exist. Their psychological reality is, however, questionable and, yet, of vital importance when working with 'real' clients. The notion of language impairment is based on the premise that something is different in the functioning of the specific linguistic systems when compared with those of 'normal' linguistic systems. The notion of a linguistic system, in turn, derives from the formal, theoretical approach to linguistics (Chapter 2) where structural properties of language are described. A specific language impairment therefore constitutes a problem in the acquisition or the functioning of the specific linguistic system. For one then to be able to ascertain that a specific problem exists, one needs to be able to determine that a problem derives from lack of structures or from unusual functioning of the structures in that system. As has been pointed out by Leonard (1987), and others, the underlying causes of specific language impairments are not always understood and therefore diagnosis may often be solely motivated by comparisons of structural patterns with 'a norm'.

Assuming that language impairment is a useful, accessible construct, another problem however presents itself. The notion of formal, theoretical linguistic systems is largely based on the notion of autonomy. Linguistic systems are

Example 3 143

studied as largely independent from one another in order to explore the nature of language and language universals (Chomsky, 1965; see also Radford, 1988). Formal linguistic approaches also maintain that we must describe and understand the structural properties of languages before we can study how they are acquired or used for communication. These formal linguistic principles of structural autonomy and structural priority have been transferred to the study of language pathology and the practice of speech therapy. Language impairment has been studied in terms of fairly separate linguistic levels and the idea that one needs to work on structures before working on communication has been an aspect of speech therapy for some time now. This is not to suggest that speech pathologists work on such formal principles alone, but simply to highlight the underlying motivations and potential consequences of working within such principles at all. It also needs to be emphasized that these structural notions filtered into the domain of language pathology because of linguistics; prior to their 'linguistic revolution' speech therapists worked with more functional, integrated models of disability and therapy.

As we see it, the above theoretical linguistic notions and the practice of speech therapy can be incompatible, reflecting their differing aims. Unlike theoretical linguistics, the practical, clinical domain of speech pathology cannot afford to divorce language from communication or ignore the interrelatedness of linguistic levels in communication. It cannot successfully do the former because the very language problem manifests itself as a problem in communicating meanings. In the clinical context where one is dealing with human ability in human interaction the theoretical notion of a linguistic system has only limited value. It serves little purpose to work on clients' hypothetical linguistic systems, bringing them in line with 'normal' linguistic systems, without considering how these systems feed into the client's ability to share meanings with others. In other words, structural linguistic analysis is not an end itself but constitutes a step within a wider analysis of communicative ability. Many linguistically based clinical tools pay lip service to this functional consideration. Crystal, Fletcher and Garman (1976), for instance, have a discourse dimension in the LARSP procedure to aid interpretation of the grammatical profile. Similarly, Grunwell (1985) discussed the importance of assessing the communicative adequacy of restricted phonological systems in her phonological assessment procedure. It is not that linguists do not appreciate the importance of integrating structural and functional considerations in linguistic assessments; the problem arises in the lack of knowledge we have of how the different levels relate to one another and thus linguistically based procedures tend only to emphasise the importance of integration without having too much to offer at the practical level. It is thus paramount that clinical linguistic approaches start to examine more seriously the links between linguistic structures and their functional roles. Fortunately, theoretical linguistic study has moved from the formal paradigm into a more functional one (e.g. Dik, 1978, Halliday, 1985) and this has started to filter into clinical linguistic approaches, albeit slowly.

Formal, structural analyses have their place in the clinical management of communication disorders. They enable one to ascertain (if based on truly representative samples obtained in a variety of contexts, over several sessions) what linguistic structures the client has at his/her disposal for achieving communicative ends. The usual approach is to change the client's system so that it becomes more like the corresponding adult or child system. Assuming that several structural components are concurrently missing from a particular system, the question arises of what to target first in remediation. In relation to children, one is often advised to follow the normal developmental pattern (Crystal, Fletcher and Garman, 1976, Grunwell, 1985). It is however noted that this may not always be the most sensible approach, given that following a normal developmental pattern may be the very problem a child is experiencing (Crystal, Fletcher and Garman, 1976). Also, following such a pattern might do very little for making the child more intelligible to other people. It may be that improving intelligibility is a top priority in treatment in order to end the child's social isolation. It may also be that this particular child learns in a different manner from others or has individual strengths which render a theoretically 'later' sound

Example 3 145

or structure more teachable. It is at the point when clinicians are identifying meaningful treatment goals that functional evaluations of structural linguistic analysis are seriously considered. The consideration of how the client's problems with linguistic structures may contribute towards communicative problems gains added significance in the context of disorders where the client cannot be expected to (re)learn a complete adult/child linguistic system. The question of how to maximize the client's limited linguistic potential to achieve personal and communicative goals becomes paramount in such circumstances. This is one type of interaction of linguistic structures and functional considerations which is of importance in the clinical context.

The interaction of linguistic levels can also be examined from the point of view of the interdependence of the levels themselves. Clinicians are only able to retain a view of language problems as isolated events because of their policy of discharging clients once the most apparent speech or language difficulty is resolved. Later educational difficulties, and indeed later emerging language problems, are thus invisible to clinicians, unless the problems are sufficiently serious to occasion re-referral. Yet, it may be these later problems which reveal most clearly how the various levels interact.

The interaction of linguistic levels gains particular significance in the assessment of linguistic skills and consequent diagnoses of problems. Interrelatedness of linguistic levels cannot be ignored because it is quite unlikely that a communication problem reflects a problem at one linguistic level alone ('pure' language impairment; Leonard, 1987, Crystal, 1987), that a problem at one level does not have an effect on other linguistic levels (e.g. Paul and Shriberg, 1982, Campbell and Shriberg, 1982, Chiat and Hirson, 1987) or that the development of specific linguistic skills is not affected by the development of other language and pragmatic skills (Donahue, 1987). Thus, a particular incorrect linguistic manifestation can be a consequence of:

1. A problem in a specific linguistic system;
2. A problem in another linguistic system than the most obvious because of interaction (e.g. absence of the

phonological contrasts reflected as lack of grammatical plurals);
3. A developmental 'trade-off' phenomenon (e.g. phonology deteriorates when syntax develops);
4. A use of a communication strategy (e.g. paraphrasing due to lack of lexical access; Chapter 3);
5. Contextual influences (e.g. inferior performance due to interactive partners; see also Example 1, above).

Considering 2–5 helps one to explore whether a linguistic problem truly exists. It appears that many clinical assessment tools designed to investigate linguistic disability tend to pay only marginal attention to the above considerations which might bring about specific linguistic structures. Concentration tends to be at one level at a time. Consequently, conclusions about linguistic ability or disability can be too readily drawn on the basis of specific aspects of linguistic performance.

Let us consider how linguistic levels can interact in the clinical context. One type of interaction is where a problem at one level appears as a problem at another level. An absence of word final fricatives in the phonological system may be reflected as lack of plurality and third person singular forms in the grammatical system. The levels of phonology and semantics can be seen interacting in that lack of phonological contrasts restricts the signalling of meanings in a lexical system (Leinonen-Davies, 1988b). Pragmatic problems often interact with linguistic skills. A client with problems in relating to other people can exhibit reduced linguistic skill simply because of lack of data. Appreciating that an apparent problem with specific skills may in fact reflect problems in other domains of communication is part of realistic clinical assessment and management.

Another type of interaction of linguistic levels has been discussed in terms of a 'trade-off' phenomenon in language development and in the context of language disability. When a child is acquiring a new structure or a language disordered individual has a problem in processing language, apparent regression in ability at one level can occur because of development or processing at another level. This is what Crystal (1987) refers to as the 'bucket' theory of language

Example 3 147

disability. In his analogy, language processing capacity is likened to a bucket.

> The bucket gets larger, as the child develops; but in the case of the language handicapped child, there is a series of holes at a certain level. As the child's language level rises, and reaches the holes, there is a stage where any extra water poured into the bucket will cause some of the water already present to overflow via the holes. An extra drop of phonology may cause an overflow of a 'drop' of syntax (p. 20).

This analogy can apply to language disability at any age.

Many studies in language development provide evidence for such 'trading-off'. For instance, when extending the length of utterances, when acquiring new words or when producing full sentences rather than isolated words phonetic and phonological accuracy has been observed to suffer (Waterson, 1978, Ingram, 1976). In this way syntax and semantics can be seen interacting with phonology and phonetics. Discourse and pragmatic factors have also been observed interacting with other levels. Crystal (1987) discusses the familiar tendency of language handicapped children to get into linguistic difficulties when telling a story as compared with producing isolated sentences. Other pragmatic influences mentioned by Crystal which are of utmost clinical importance include the effect upon other linguistic skills of such contextual factors as familiarity, task complexity and distribution of information in utterances (also, Campbell and Shriberg, 1982). Therefore, one is not to assume too readily that the lack of linguistic structures in the client's productive language or gaps in his/her understanding are necessarily indicative of lack of linguistic skill.

Considering the interaction of linguistic levels amongst themselves and in relation to pragmatics is important in a clinical pragmatic approach to language disability which aims to understand how communicative occurrences come into being and aims to facilitate the emergence of appropriate ones. Currently available assessment tools encourage clinicians to analyse performance at the various linguistic levels quite independently. Most clinicians will add to linguistic assessments their findings from observational assessment of the client's ability to interact with others. One hears less about the interaction between form, content and use, or about the interaction between linguistic levels. This is probably because frameworks for describing these in a systematic manner are not available rather than because clinicians regard these issues as unimportant. Treatment can also suffer from the separation of linguistic levels (Chapter 7). It is quite possible that positive interactions occur between levels so that improvements in pragmatic skills improve phonological and syntactic performance or that an enlarging vocabulary will lead to better pragmatic performance through a growth of confidence.

Some guidelines are beginning to emerge. Leinonen-Davies (1988a) considered the interaction of phonology and lexicon with the view to providing some guidelines for phonological therapy focusing on the notions of interaction and functionality. She suggests that phonological contrasts can be chosen for remediation in terms of their potential detrimental effect on the signalling of meaning differences in the lexicon and potentially in communication. She provides some guidelines as to which phonological contrasts are potentially most damaging for children's lexicons and thus, logically, most motivating to tackle in remediation. Leinonen (1991) also considers how actual assessment of phonology can take into account such interaction. She suggests an approach to phonological process analysis which from the outset focuses on functionality, contrasting with approaches where functionality is more of an 'after-thought' than an initial motivation. A functional approach to phonological therapy is based on the notion that phonological development is functionally motivated; that children learn phonological systems to serve communicative ends (Leinonen, 1990). The scope of the current volume does not merit a more detailed account here. This simply serves to highlight that work recognizing the importance of interaction of linguistic levels in clinical linguistic tools is in progress, albeit on a rather limited and modest scale. We believe that the field of clinical linguistics has a great deal more to offer to the practising clinician if it begins to address seriously the issues of functionality and interaction.

Chapter 5

Disturbance of pragmatic functioning

The speech pathology profession has recognized for some time a group of people who have trouble communicating with others despite adequate ability to produce structurally well-formed language. Such people may talk incessantly or be silent when a contribution is expected; they may give the impression that the social situation has been misconstrued or they may, in some other way, render their communicative partner uncomfortable. Not only the communicative partners but also the person concerned may become aware that interactions are not proceeding as they expect or intend. Speech acts are not being successfully performed because the right things are not being said in the right way at the right time and because the implications of what is said by either party are not fully understood by at least one of the participants. A problem of pragmatics can be said to exist in such situations.

This type of communication difficulty is encountered by individuals with a variety of diagnostic backgrounds. It may be encountered by people who have received head injury or a stroke, even though, superficially, their language production and comprehension abilities appear normal (Code, 1987). In children similar difficulties can occur. Pragmatic problems are usually noticed in middle childhood, sometimes after superficially successful resolution of language acquisition problems. Such problems are currently referred to by clinicians as difficulties arising from a 'semantic-pragmatic disorder' (Rapin and Allen, 1983). We shall argue in this chapter that such problems could be more appropriately referred to as problems of pragmatic

competence or performánce (mobilization of this competence) associated with certain factors within the client or
the client's environment. As will become apparent from the
review of literature, those labelled as semantic-pragmatic
disordered form rather a heterogeneous population; the
real problems of such individuals can become masked by
an all-encompassing diagnostic label. We shall suggest a
way of conceptualizing communication problems which
highlights the idiosyncracy of individuals' problems while
recognizing the existence of a domain of problems which
can be said to be pragmatic in nature.

LITERATURE REVIEW

Children who appear to have problems with language use
and appropriate communicative behaviour have been discussed in the literature well before the coining of the term
'semantic-pragmatic disorder'. Fraser and Blockley (1973),
for instance, described children who had difficulty in gen-
erating appropriate new utterances on the basis of taught
language forms, possibly because of conceptual and perceptual difficulties. They were noted to have serious difficulties with respect to relationships in space and time.
The major underlying problems for these children were
thought to concern conceptualizations rather than linguistic
knowledge and skills. These children appear to exhibit
communication problems which could be described as both
semantic and pragmatic in nature. Currently, the term
semantic-pragmatic disorder is primarily used to refer to
children with adequate linguistic skills whose problems lie
in the areas of comprehension and appropriate language
use. The terms 'high level language disorder' and 'conversational disability' are also sometimes used to describe
these impairments.

Lucas (1980) employs the terms 'semantic' and 'pragmatic'
in the context of 'language disordered' children, whose
main problems seem to lie in the use rather than structure
of language. Lucas makes a connection between underlying
semantic disorder and pragmatic problems which ensue.
The occurrence of the following manifestations, singly or

in combinations, is considered symptomatic of a language disorder (presumably a semantic disorder):

1. Inadequate acquisition of the perceptual and functional characteristics of objects, actions, events.
2. Inability to relate the lexicon with objects, actions or events.
3. Failure to acquire the semantic rules underlying speech acts. Social or pragmatic rules are not specified since the disorder in that case would not be one of language.

In the section discussing 'specific semantic disorders' the following (further) characteristics are included: auditory misperception; off-target responding; tangentiality; syntactic error; semantic word errors; word-finding problems; neologisms; problems in identifying topics and referents; echolalia; and verbal perseveration.

Moving toward discussion of pragmatic problems Lucas states that whenever a semantic disorder occurs, particularly when this affects a child's perception and interpretation of semantic relations in the environment, a pragmatic problem ensues. For Lucas, a pragmatic disorder exists when a child is not effective in conveying intents.

A child may be considered ineffective in performing speech acts when the child:

1. physically attempts to solve situational problems better suited to verbal solutions;
2. never initiates verbalizations to meet specific needs;
3. inappropriately cues the hearer with inadequate paralinguistic cues and/or
4. lacks the ability to specify referents (p. 109).

Further behavioural manifestations which might indicate pragmatic problems would be: waiting to be given what is needed rather than making requests; using inappropriate paralinguistic and prosodic features and uncooperative behaviour.

Lucas considers semantic and pragmatic aspects of one's communicative functioning to be closely linked. As will be argued later in this chapter, this does not necessarily need to be the case. Furthermore, as the above definition of pragmatic disorder suggests, the investigation of pragmatic problems focuses primarily on speech act performance. In the more specific discussion of the behavioural manifestations indicative of ineffective performance of speech acts, Lucas does however appear to consider issues of presupposition and informativity too. Lucas' discussion also suggests a direct relationship between surface manifestations and the notion of disorder. What may appear in surface communicative behaviour may result from a variety of within-client and outside-client influences, and therefore great care needs to be taken in the employment of the term 'disorder' which is not only client-focused but also medically motivated (see further below). In a later work Lucas Arwood (1983) stresses that adults frequently accept too much responsibility during interactions with language handicapped children. When this is the case (e.g. when the adult always initiates), it is impossible to judge the child's capacity for the performance of speech acts.

Rapin and Allen (1983) introduced the term 'semantic-pragmatic deficit syndrome' as part of their sub-categorization of developmental language disability (DLD) in children. DLD covers a wide range of problems which can cluster in specific ways reflecting more specific impairments. Although, theoretically speaking, almost any combination of problems can be found, Rapin and Allen identified certain frequently occurring combinations. Two of the six sub-categories involved pragmatic problems.

> Children with *syntactic-pragmatic syndrome* (italics by the current authors) show grossly impaired syntax and severely limited pragmatic use of language. Comprehension of connected discourse and of the demands of interpersonal conversation are also impaired (p. 176).

Similar comprehension and communication problems are evidenced in the group of children with the *semantic-pragmatic syndrome*, with the exception that their language is structurally well formed. The main difficulty with these children lies in the 'encod(ing) of meaning relevant to the conversational situation' (p. 174). Rapin and Allen also consider the difficulty of determining whether the seemingly irrelevant responses of these children reflect psychotic disturbance (e.g. thought disorder).

Rapin and Allen (1987) revise the subcategorizations. The syntactic-pragmatic syndrome is excluded with the addition of the *lexical-syntactic deficit syndrome*. Even though the name of this category might not suggest association with pragmatic problems, such children were observed to experience difficulties in formulating connected language, especially within the constraints of conversation. Additional pragmatic problems include avoidance of initiations in conversations and difficulty in giving a coherent account of prior incidents. The distinguishing characteristic of this syndrome is severe word retrieval deficit (anomia). While the defining characteristics of the semantic-pragmatic deficit syndrome remain the same, further details of behavioural manifestations are given. Such children are said to misinterpret what is said to them, responding to literal meanings and to key words rather than what is actually meant. Many are echolalic, some perseverate or talk excessively. The semantic difficulties are said to involve semantic paraphasia and lack of semantic specificity. The difficulty of determining whether problems are 'semantic' or 'pragmatic' in nature needs however to be borne in mind (see later discussion).

By identifying specific clusterings of behaviour characteristics in the sub-categorization of the types of 'language disorders', Rapin and Allen highlight the heterogeneous nature of communication problems. The term 'deficit syndrome' captures the idea of the clustering of disabilities in contrast to the term 'disorder' which suggests a more specifiable entity.

Rapin and Allen (1987) also discuss the relationship between the 'semantic-pragmatic deficit syndrome' and autism. By stating that 'the semantic-pragmatic deficit syndrome is frequently seen in verbal autistic children' (p. 25), Rapin and Allen make it clear that what is under discussion is a cluster of surface manifestations. In other words, they do not presuppose a condition termed 'semantic-pragmatic disorder' which would be clearly distinguished from autism. Rather, children with the semantic-pragmatic deficit syndrome, with or without autism, share behaviour characteristics with those with autism, however, exhibiting more 'severe' symptoms of pragmatic disturbance. In this way, the fuzziness of borderlines is acknowledged (cf. Bishop, 1989). The relationship between pragmatic problems and autism will be explored further in relation to a conceptualization of pragmatic knowledge later in this chapter.

In one of the most widely used texts in 'clinical pragmatics' (Gallagher and Prutting, 1983), Prutting and Kirchner divide pragmatic problems in language disordered children into, essentially, three groups.

1. There are children who appear to lack sensitivity to the various dimensions of social context.
2. There are children whose cognitive deficit places a boundary on their communicative potential by restricting vocabulary and limiting comprehension. These limitations may interfere with the ability to establish and maintain topics, identify and signal referents and make appropriate lexical choices.
3. There are children whose inability to handle linguistic structuring at the discourse level interferes with coherent, reciprocal communication, even though they may be aware of and sensitive to what is required.

These categorizations draw attention to the variable nature of pragmatic deficits. They highlight potential differences in the underlying causes of inappropriate communicative behaviours. These underlying constructs may be social, cognitive or linguistic in nature. We believe that this conceptualization of pragmatic problems is useful, recognizing that what presents itself as an underlying 'pragmatic disorder' may in fact stem from some other type of underlying problem. We shall pursue this further in our conceptualization of the notion 'semantic-pragmatic' disorder.

In the same edited volume Fey and Leonard (1983) tentatively identified three patterns of conversational participation in language impaired children.

1. Unwillingness or inability to engage in conversation and general unresponsiveness relative to normal children of the same age.
2. Participation in conversation but with frequent use of

back channel behaviours which maintain the topic without adding new information to it. These minimal responses serve to maintain social contact but enable the child to avoid taking the floor. Children exhibiting this pattern can be described as responsive but non-assertive.
3. Normal initiating and responding behaviour albeit with impaired linguistic performance.

Children in group 1

may be regarded as having general pragmatic impairments since their unwillingness or inability to engage in conversations has a profound influence in all areas of language use (p. 77).

Children exhibiting pattern two were thought to have selective, rather than general pragmatic impairments in that their problems in production and comprehension of syntax lead to non-assertive behaviour. They may make few requests for clarification; have a restricted range of lexical substitutions with which to respond to others' clarification requests; have a restricted repertoire of speech acts and a limited range of linguistic forms with which to operate and perform. They may also have problems in using anaphoric pronouns to encode previously established referents. Children in group 3 can be thought of as exhibiting linguistic impairment without severe pragmatic consequences. They could however exhibit such unusual behaviours as over-reliance on non-verbal means of communication.

Although Friel-Patti and Conti-Ramsden (1984) did not set out to discuss the concept of semantic-pragmatic disorder, much of what they have to say impinges on the concept, therefore selective portions of their important contribution to the understanding of disturbed communicative development are summarized. Friel-Patti and Conti-Ramsden draw attention to the diversity of sub-types of language impairment. They state that

studies with either loose or different criteria of language impairment often produced conflicting results. Studies with strictly defined criteria may yield results that are not easily generalized to the population of language impaired children (p. 169).

Given this difficult situation they caution that our knowledge concerning discourse development in atypical language learners is clouded. A recurring problem is that many language-impaired children appear to function at a level somewhere between that of MLU-matched children and age-matched children. Therefore it is difficult to form a picture of whether cognitive, social or linguistic factors most affect their performance. Furthermore, many of them are found to have deficits in non-linguistic representational skills which could affect their discourse performance. Hypothesizing a variety of different language sub-skills, Friel-Patti and Conti-Ramsden find that studies, including their own, suggest that communicative and structural aspects of language involve different abilities. The studies they consider also seem to indicate that the sub-skills involved in pragmatic and discourse functioning are heterogeneous and separate, drawing attention to the possibility that unpopularity with peers and with adults may contribute to lack of social knowledge in some children, and that this in turn may inhibit pragmatic development. These authors also suggest that certain language-impaired children have difficulties with types of discourse other than conversation and that such difficulties may be related to cognition in very specific ways. It was also pointed out that these types of difficulty may well persist throughout the school years.

Adams and Bishop (1989) compared a group of 14 'semantic-pragmatic disordered' children (aged 8 to 12 years) with 43 other language-impaired children (aged 8 to 12 years) and 67 control children (aged 4 to 12 years), with the aim of finding an objective characterization of semantic-pragmatic disorder. A further aim was to discover whether reliable and useful information could be provided by analysis of short semi-structured interactions. Acknowledging that the variability of topic in natural conversation could lead to variable performance not attributable to the child's ability, Adams and Bishop decided to rely on five- to ten-minute adult-controlled conversations centering around a set of photographs. The data was analysed in terms of exchange structure, turntaking, repairs and cohesion (proforms and demonstratives). The children given the label 'semantic-pragmatic disorder' were observed to produce more initiations than the other children and this was considered 'a stable and abnormal conversational characteristic' (p. 238). Trends for violating turns by interrupting and for use of unestablished reference were also observed. Adequate inter-rater reliability was obtained, suggesting that the data was sufficient and that certain conversational characteristics led to a diagnosis of semantic-pragmatic disorder. Adams and Bishop acknowledge the circularity of the research method which first classifies children on an impressionistic basis and then assesses those aspects of behaviour thought to have created that impression. However, this is regarded as 'a necessary first step towards divising more rigorous and objective criteria for classification' (p. 213). Ideally, this will lead to more refined sub-categorization of pragmatic problems. A further point concerns the ages of control children: had younger age groups been included it seems possible that some of the abnormal behaviours of the children identified as semantic-pragmatic disordered might have matched those of the younger controls. A companion paper by Bishop and Adams (1989) which focuses on listener judgements of pragmatic inappropriacy is also of interest here, but will be discussed in Chapter 6 in relation to issues in assessment. What needs to be noted here, however, is that the semantic-pragmatic disordered children tended to provide the listener with too much or too little information for processing of data.

Several studies based on individual cases of semantic-pragmatic disorder have emerged. The focus tends to be on identifying inappropriate communicative behaviours which are 'pragmatic in nature'. These behaviour characteristics are then assumed to reflect some underlying 'semantic pragmatic disorder'. McTear (1985c) describes the communicative behaviour of a ten-year-old boy in detail, using an approach derived from discourse and conversational analyses. The boy has received treatment for an 'articulation problem' and has marked suprasegmental problems (e.g. is observed to speak over-loudly). Grammatical structures are reported to be unproblematic. Occasional confusions with temporal sequencing and the perception of cause and effect are also observed. Eye contact is described as poor and he does not face his communicative partner. He also physically separates himself from groups. He has some motor abnormalities, perceptual disturbances and 'restrictions of the imagination'. Detailed analysis of the boy's interactional and discourse manifestations revealed a tendency for literal interpretation, minimal conversational contributions, failure to use ellipsis, difficulty in making factual, and especially causal, information clear, frequent use of 'I don't know', failure to take his partner's knowledge into account or failure to differentiate between his own and other people's knowledge. Inferencing also appeared difficult for this child, though it is uncertain to what extent this may be due to limited knowledge of the world.

McTear concludes that the 'bizarre and confused' impression created by this ten-year-old boy results from four main causes: deficiencies in handling and integrating information; uncertainty of the knowledge possessed by others; overuse of coping strategies and shortage of non-threatening experiences in which coping strategies may be unnecessary. These conclusions are valuable in many ways. They are particularly valuable in highlighting how apparently disparate communicative behaviours may have common underlying causes (even though these causes are ultimately hypothetical) and in recognizing that inappropriate or unsuccessful communication does not necessarily entail an underlying 'disorder' but may reflect one's attempts at coping with communication problems (Communication strategies, Chapter 3).

The response to McTear's (1985b) assertion that the way forward in the study of semantic-pragmatic disorders would be through detailed case studies and rigorous and extensive analyses of language samples, Conti-Ramsden and Gunn (1986) presented a detailed case study of the boy Tony together with a summary of the therapy regime which had been offered to him throughout the period of the study. This particular child demonstrated many of the difficulties mentioned by other writers in the field but not all of them. Conti-Ramsden and Gunn therefore ask whether individual children will demonstrate a selection of problems drawn from a similar broad range; whether therapy affects the form in which the syndrome is demonstrated or whether the picture of the disorder is likely to be reliably different at different developmental stages. It was also found that Tony's communicative behaviour altered over time in several respects and that many of his observed difficulties were not revealed (were concealed even) by the usual range of language assessments. For this reason Conti-Ramsden and Gunn recommend that investigations aspire to the depth of detail advocated by McTear but with the breadth illustrated by their own study. The value of longitudinal studies is particularly stressed.

Papers on semantic-pragmatic disorder written by clinicians with daily contact with this population are beginning to emerge (Culloden, Hyde-Wright and Shipman, 1986, Jones, Smedly and Jennings, 1986, Smedly, 1989, Spence, Fleetwood, Geliot, Wrench, Earles and Searby, 1989). They constitute valuable observational accounts of behavioural manifestations of these children. Even though lacking in rigour, they demonstrate the range of problems encountered by these children and the difficulties involved in treatment. An accessible account of 'conversational disability' aimed primarily at teachers is provided by Beveridge and Conti-Ramsden (1987).

Problematic communicative (pragmatic) manifestations can clearly stem from a variety of causes. Literature on many different types of primary deficits has reported resultant problems in pragmatic functioning. In such instances, the term 'pragmatic disorder' is not appropriate, given the possibility that individuals with no known primary deficit can nevertheless exhibit similar problematic behaviours.

Bryan (1988) drew attention to studies of right hemisphere damage in adults with subsequent difficulties in 'lexical-semantic and high level language processing' possibly with accompanying 'spatial, perceptual and emotional problems'. Difficulties were found in speech act comprehension, comprehension of non-literal meanings, appreciation of metaphors, humour, connotative aspects of meaning and paralinguistic cues. There was insensitivity to the pragmatic aspects of meaning and failure to use contextual information to derive meaning or to extract and isolate key elements, to see the relationships among them, to integrate them into an over-all structure and to draw inferences based on these relationships, both in complex linguistic tasks and in discourse. Bryan points out that Weintraub and Mesulam (1983) not surprisingly suggest that early damage to the right hemisphere causes profound impairment in the development of those skills described above. Bryan also discusses emotional and interpersonal difficulties which may be associated with right hemisphere damage or with the specific language problems resulting from it. If there is indeed a neurologically based syndrome appropriately labelled semantic/pragmatic, it would appear on the basis of these studies likely that some form of right hemisphere impairment is involved or possibly impaired connection between right and left hemisphere.

Hawkins (1989) draws particular attention to the observation that some aphasic patients appear to have problems at the level of discourse rather than at any other level. He uses the term 'discourse aphasia' in this connection. This view is in contrast to that of Ulatowska and Bond (1983) who found discourse skills such as narrating and providing information about procedures (e.g. How do we make tea?) relatively unimpaired.

The assumption that a pragmatic component of the communicative competence exists separately from other aspects of one's communicative knowledge is evident in the above studies. The question of what this 'pragmatic component' might entail will be considered later on in this chapter. When a person is regarded as having a 'pure pragmatic deficit', presumably only this pragmatic component is being affected. It is particularly difficult to determine the differential status of such a component given that 'pragmatics' concerns appropriate social interaction. Johnston (1985) explores possible differences between deficits in social cognition and 'true pragmatic disorder' (p. 90).

Donahue's (1987) discussion of the relationship between linguistic and pragmatic development in learning-disabled children is based on the assumption that syntax and pragmatics are separable. Given Curtiss' (1977, 1981) studies on autism and the case of Genie, it indeed appears that selective aspects of one's communicative functioning can be affected, thus suggesting 'a modular theory of mind'. Within this premise Donahue discusses three propositions.

1. Learning disabled children's syntactic-semantic knowledge is unrelated to their pragmatic competence.
2. Learning disabled children's syntactic-semantic knowledge constrains their pragmatic competence.
3. Learning disabled children's pragmatic competence constrains their syntactic-semantic knowledge.

While she comes to the over-all conclusion that it is not possible on the basis of current research, and is probably unwise to attempt, to rule out possible hypotheses generated by each view, she considers view 1 as 'at best . . . counterintuitive' (p. 129), view 2 'the most intuitively obvious position' (p. 146) and view 3 'the most speculative position' even though 'it has great potential for accounting for individual routes to linguistic and pragmatic development' (p. 169). Donahue further suggests that indeed it may be unnecessary to try to draw conclusions about these views since they can be considered 'equally viable explanations for different subgroups of LD (learning disabled)' rather than competing hypothesis. She also gives a timely reminder that Steckol (1983) suggested certain inappropriate language therapy formats as one possible source of linguistic-pragmatic discrepancies. Theoretical investigation of the relations of different types of knowledge is particularly important in the context of communication, and more specifically pragmatic, disorders, if the field is to move from descriptions of behaviour characteristics to understanding the nature of the problems.

In their discussion of the development of linguistic communication in association with mental retardation, Abbeduto and Rosenberg (1987) also indicate that such skills as turn taking, recognizing and fulfilling obligations established by illocutionary acts (e.g. a question requires an answer), active participation in conversation and the co-ordination of propositional content and contextual information when performing illocutionary acts are not completely predictable from an individual's level of linguistic competence or non-verbal or cognitive maturity. They further explore influences which can affect the acquisition and functioning of pragmatic knowledge. Two major types of influences are discussed: environmental factors and 'supporting competences', which include communicatively relevant linguistic, cognitive and social abilities and knowledge bases. The ability to inference and knowledge about social conventions and the world support communicative functioning. Additionally, it is assumed that pragmatic rules enable speakers to match their intended message with appropriate linguistic expression and social context. Such rules are assumed to be part of a person's 'linguistic communicative competence'. This conceptualization of communicative functioning takes an integrative view of communication, recognizing the various factors which shape the acquisition and use of communicative knowledge. These issues will be explored later on in this chapter.

'Semantic-pragmatic disorder', being manifested in inappropriate social and communicative behaviour, shares many features with other childhood problems, namely autism and Asperger's syndrome (see also childhood psychosis, below). The question of where to place the boundaries between these conditions, or indeed whether they can be delineated, has been discussed notably by Rapin and Allen (1987), Howlin (1987), Wing (1988), Bishop and Rosenbloom (1987) and Bishop (1989). Several suggestions as to the nature of the relationship exist. Rapin and Allen's study suggests that 'semantic-pragmatic disorder' and autism can be co-occurring conditions, both having the potential for disturbance in verbal and non-verbal social behaviour. The differentiating factor could be that of severity of disturbance, autism exhibiting more extreme cases of communicative abnormality and Asperger's syndrome (Wing, 1988) and semantic-pragmatic disorder milder forms of inappropriacy. Wing suggests that autism and Asperger's syndrome fall on an 'autistic continuum' by showing impairment in three main areas of social function: deficits in social recognition, social communication and social understanding. In regard to this point, Bishop (1989) suggests that the differences between the two lie not only in the severity of social impairment but also in pattern of symptoms. More specifically, Bishop differentiates autism, Asperger's syndrome and semantic-pragmatic disorder in terms of social and language impairment. According to Bishop, autistic children have persisting deficits in both;

children with Asperger's syndrome have no appreciable language problems but present themselves as clumsy and socially inept and those with semantic-pragmatic problems present early language delay with persisting communicative problems. However, while recognizing the overlap, Bishop considers it clearer to keep the two conditions separate, diagnosing autistic only those children who fit conventional diagnostic critera (Rutter, 1989; American Psychiatric Association, 1987). Semantic-pragmatic disorder is differentiated from autism by using the term for

> children who are not autistic but who initially present with a picture of language delay and receptive language impairment and who then learn to speak clearly and in complex sentences, with semantic and pragmatic abnormalities becoming increasingly obvious as their verbal proficiency increases (p. 118).

Bishop also draws attention to the fact that diagnosis of autism should be based on behaviour before five years of age. Semantic-pragmatic problems, on the other hand, tend not to be taken seriously until well after that stage. Such children might also have been diagnosed as suffering from Asperger's syndrome, sharing 'milder' characteristics of communicative disturbance with this group.

Referring to these groups of children as sharing commonality in deficit is a clinically well-motivated enterprise in terms of planning and administering of treatment. However, it does not seem particularly helpful to attribute a common feature of autism to the syndromes. While Bishop's categorization of the three conditions in relation to both social and language impairment is interesting, one must not rule out the theoretical possibility that pragmatic disturbance may exist without language disability, even though pragmatic disturbance would almost inevitably interfere with language development in some way (Donahue, 1987; above). It may also be the case that pragmatically disturbed children in whom semantic problems are still evident, despite the resolution of other linguistic difficulties, are the ones who become referred to speech therapy. Furthermore, the very nature of the profession of speech and language therapy may attract principally children whose pragmatic

problems are allied to semantic and other linguistic difficulties. If such a selective population provides the data
for research, the definition of semantic-pragmatic disorder
is largely predetermined. Indeed, one may question the
appropriacy of the term 'high level language disorder' in
this context, given that pragmatic disturbance may not
always be closely allied to language. The varied nature of
pragmatic disturbances will be explored shortly.

Approaching semantic, pragmatic and other communication problems from a non-speech pathology viewpoint,
Hassibi and Breuer (1980) focus on the need to differentiate
between psychotic and language disordered children. The
language disorder of most concern to them is 'aphasia',
whereas some features which might lead one now to consider 'semantic-pragmatic disorder' were discussed by them
at that time as possibly 'psychotic'. The psychotic child is
described as one whose speech is low in communicative
value because of disregard for the needs of the listener.

> His communicative skills may be underdeveloped in that
> he does not comprehend that words must have shared
> meanings in order to be understood, and their temporal
> orders must reflect the relational order between things
> and events. He may use pronouns without having pro-
> vided the reference . . . he may even condense several
> words together to make a neologism (pp. 135–136).

The children convey the impression of being unable to
see themselves in a variety of roles, report on their past
or present feelings or to form opinions about their relationships with others. Further description of the psychotic
child's communicative behaviour deals with the more emotional and imaginative aspects of their disturbance which
could well affect pragmatic performance without semantic
deficit. Such features would include wandering attention
and the introduction of unrelated elements connected with
interior rather than with shared themes and with the child's
'chaotic experiences' and 'anomalous picture of reality'.
Topic tends to be determined by the child's threatening
vision of forces beyond his/her control and the inability to
escape from imaginary enemies. Strategies even when the
child is in control are limited to destruction and intimida-

tion. Accounts of dreams and daydreams may reawaken the intolerable feelings associated with them, more especially for the child who finds it difficult to distinguish between what is taking place in conceptual or in actual reality.

Given that the behavioural manifestations of children diagnosed as 'psychotic' or 'semantic-pragmatic disordered' can be similar, there is a danger of misguided diagnosis. It is helpful to encounter the perspective of a profession other than one's own when seeking to understand a complex problem, and we feel that while all the professions concerned with childhood communication problems could benefit from one anothers' expertise, there is a special case for increased co-operation between psychiatrists and speech pathologists where 'semantic-pragmatic disorders' and childhood psychoses are concerned.

Finally, McTear (1985b) observed that while the understanding of disabilities in the use of language had increased in the previous ten years due to an increase in publications, lack of theoretical rigour could be seen in the lack of an explanatory theory of the relationship between pragmatic disability and language development and in lack of terminological and organizational consistency. With or without rigour, it is still the case that we lack a single, unifying explanatory theory of the kind that McTear and others have sought. What is lacking is a rigorous exploration of what constitutes pragmatic disability: such exploration is logical prior to examining the relationship of disability to development. One firstly needs a clear conception of the variables which one is then to compare.

THE PRAGMATIC COMPONENT OF COMMUNICATIVE COMPETENCE

The issues concerning the notion of 'semantic-pragmatic' disorder can be explored further in relation to the notion of communicative competence. In line with Saussure's previously conceived terms of *'la langue'* and *'le parole'*, Chomsky (1965) distinguishes underlying knowledge of linguistic structures from the actual linguistic performance. The assumption is that one cannot perform linguistically without competence, while lack of performance does not presume lack of competence. While retaining Chomsky's distinction between competence and performance, Hymes (1972a) pointed out that for one to be able to communicate in culturally and contextually appropriate ways knowledge other than linguistic is required. This knowledge was termed 'communicative competence'. Schiefelbusch (1984, 5) summarizes the concept of communicative competence as

> the totality of experience-driven knowledge and skill that enables a speaker to produce utterances that are structurally well-formed, referentially accurate, and socially appropriate in culturally determined communication contexts, and to understand the speech of others as a joint function of structural characteristics and social context.

The term communicative competence can be perceived as a cover term for all types of knowledge required for communication to be possible and successful. It can be perceived as consisting of 'sectors'(Hymes, 1972a, 281; also Faerch and Kasper, 1984, 214) or components, namely linguistic, non-verbal and pragmatic (including social and cultural norms; see below) which provide the underlying communicative potential. The mobilization of this potential rests upon cognitive, motor, perceptual, emotional and contextual factors which bear upon individuals and interactive contexts. They not only shape the final manifestations of the underlying competences but also affect the initial acquisition of the knowledge and experience constituting communicative competence.

Underlying appropriate communicative behaviour, be it productive or receptive, must lie some knowledge of how, where and when to behave in a particular manner. Such knowledge can be assumed to consist of 'knowing that' and 'knowing how' components (Faerch and Kasper, 1984). This model was developed with the practical purpose of understanding the role of pragmatic knowledge in speech production and reception, in language acquisition and learning and, in particular, with the purpose of shedding light on the potential effects of the classroom environment and the pragmatic knowledge of one's first language on the learning of pragmatic principles in another language. Since the second language learner and the person encountering communication problems, for whatever other reasons, have parallels, the 'Faerch and Kasper' model has relevance in the communication pathology context. The parallel is that of encountering a problem in communication due to lack of knowledge. One must not however forget that second language learners have many advantages over a communicatively handicapped individual. They already possess much linguistic and pragmatic knowledge which functions adequately in a specific language community or specific culture and therefore have already demonstrated ability to learn and function; they have a point of comparison to help when a communication problem is encountered; they know they are able and need not think whether they are able; they may doubt their ability to learn or use a foreign language but they can draw comfort from the knowledge that they have once successfully mastered most of the skills involved.

Two types of communicatively relevant knowledge are distinguished: declarative knowledge = *'knowledge that'* and procedural knowledge = *'knowledge how'*. These are defined by Faerch and Kasper (1984, 215) as follows.

Declarative knowledge: 'taxonomic', 'static', comprises, for instance, an individual's knowledge of the rules and elements of one or more language(s), not related to specific communicative goals or language use in real time; is divided into different but interrelated components . . .

Procedural knowledge: process-oriented, 'dynamic', selects and combines parts of declarative knowledge for the purpose of reaching specific communicative goals, observing constraints imposed by language processing in real time (sequencing, processing capacity of the speaker/hearer).

Faerch and Kasper state that in terms of cognitive psychology, declarative pragmatic knowledge is considered non-automatized and conscious while procedural pragmatic knowledge is assumed automatized and unconscious. We find this confusing since it appears likely that declarative

and procedural pragmatic knowledge can both exist in conscious or unconscious form depending on context and/or
level of development. If this were true it would crucially
affect teaching methods and therapeutic approaches since
attempts to teach awareness of that which is normally unconscious might be non-facilitative.

According to Faerch and Kasper, 'pragmatically relevant
declarative knowledge' includes the following:

1. Knowledge of the linguistic structure of a language; of
   the rules and items at phonological, syntactic and lexical
   levels. This knowledge provides a verbal means of expressing meanings in communication. This knowledge
   is also assumed to include specification of the communicative potential of linguistic elements and structures.
2. Knowledge of the possible speech acts in specific socio-
   cultural settings and the conditions underlying speech
   act performance (e.g. Searle, 1969; Chapter 3).
3. Knowledge about the ways in which speech acts can be
   combined to form coherent discourse. This constitutes
   knowledge about structural characteristics of discourse
   genres: of exchange structure; of opening and closing
   sequences; of external modification of speech acts (e.g.
   how to use a presequence to modify the impact of a
   refusal).
4. Knowledge about socio-cultural values, norms and
   institutions. This includes knowledge about conversational maxims (Grice, 1975) and other interactional
   principles such as face-saving devices.
5. Knowledge about the features in the context which are
   relevant for the production of communicatively appropriate occurrences or for interpretation. This includes
   knowledge about the relationships between individuals
   and the setting.
6. Knowledge about the world. This includes knowledge
   about facts, objects, and relations (e.g. cause-effect).
   This appears to include knowledge which is more
   general than that covered in 1–5.

It appears not to suffice to possess declarative knowledge
only; one needs to be able to select and combine parts of

this knowledge to reach communicative goals, in accordance with the constraints of language processing. According to Faerch and Kasper's definition of pragmatic 'knowledge how', this knowledge component selects and combines relevant declarative knowledge with the purpose of reaching specific communicative goals. In order to distinguish this knowledge component from cognitive processing, it may be more appropriate to assume that 'the knowing how' *informs* the process of selection and integration of declarative knowledge.

Three aspects of procedural knowledge are discussed by Faerch and Kasper. The first aspect involves goal-formulation as determined by the outcome of context analysis. That is to say that communication has a purpose or a goal which is determined in relation to what has occurred previously in the interaction, whom one is interacting with, one's needs and circumstances etc. For instance, one's goal may be to make a relevant comment on an already mentioned topic. The specification of the goal involves matching knowledge of the communicative situation with one's intention and speech act knowledge. Having decided what one is aiming to achieve the second step is to choose the linguistic expression most likely to fulfil the specified intention. This phase is referred to as verbal planning. Since it may be that the most appropriate expression will be a non-verbal one or even a zero expression, the 'verbal planning' phase may be considered in more general terms (given that the notion of pragmatics is considered in a wider sense than linguistic pragmatics in the current volume). This planning phase then involves matching appropriate expression with context and intent. The third procedural stage involves monitoring execution. A specific aspect of this is that of monitoring the feedback provided by one's interlocutors. This feedback is then fed into the procedural mechanism, affecting subsequent goal formulation and matching of expression with intent.

Within this general framework we can explore the notion of pragmatic knowledge. The six types of declarative knowledge discussed by Faerch and Kasper are referred to as 'components of pragmatically relevant declarative knowledge' (p. 215). Indeed, most human knowledge is pragmatically relevant in the sense of being relevant for human communication. The question is whether knowledge exists which can be specifically referred to as pragmatic knowledge. Pragmatic knowledge concerns a speaker's knowledge of what constitutes a contextually relevant and appropriate contribution and how to combine this knowledge with one's knowledge of the means available for expression and with one's communicative purpose and intention. From the listener's point of view, pragmatic knowledge involves knowing that the speaker has an intention and that as a listener one needs to form a hypothesis of what that intention may be and to test the hypothesis in terms of its likelihood (Leech, 1983). The pragmatic knowledge component of the communicative competence can then be considered as consisting of a store of 'knowing that' and a procedural component which informs the selection and integration of this knowledge in contextually relevant and appropriate ways and in accordance with one's intention ('knowing how').

The question is, however, what exactly would such pragmatic knowledge components consist of. Diverging from Faerch and Kasper's conceptualization, a pragmatic knowledge component which is separate from one's linguistic knowledge can be assumed. The knowledge of linguistic units and the rules for combining these in a language ('linguistic knowing that and how') can be considered separate from pragmatic knowledge 'that' which involves knowledge of communicative principles (see below). Pragmatic knowledge 'how', however, accesses linguistic knowledge when matching intention with appropriate means of expression and pragmatic knowledge 'that'. Similarly, one can assume a store of knowledge of non-verbal signals and signs used in communication which also feed into the pragmatic knowledge 'how'. This conceptualization of pragmatic knowledge and linguistic (non-verbal) knowledge being separate at an underlying level is supported by the observation that linguistic disability need not necessarily imply disturbance in the pragmatic knowledge component or vice versa. Linguistic disability and problems with pragmatic knowledge can, of course, affect the acquisition or mobilization of the other knowledge component. The point is that not knowing linguistic rules does not imply lack of knowledge of pragmatic principles or vice versa.

Before examining what these pragmatic principles of 'knowing that' may be, the relationship of world, social, cultural and contextual knowledge to pragmatic knowledge needs to be considered. Is it possible, or is it necessary, to differentiate between knowledge of the facts about the world (e.g. objects; their permanence; relations), of societies and cultures (e.g. one needs to be direct or indirect in a specific culture) or of contexts (e.g. interview register) from pragmatic knowledge about communication. Knowing what the world is like provides one with common points of reference with others and provides conversational topics. Part of this world knowledge would be knowledge of objects, their defining characteristics, of cause–effect and so forth. One could also assume that this knowledge includes knowing that humans interact or communicate with one another for some purpose. This could be considered the point at which world knowledge and pragmatic knowledge border upon one another. In the communication pathology context where it is useful to consider communication as a phenomenon with unity and coherence any knowledge about the dynamics of communication can be considered as aspects of one type of knowledge, termed pragmatic knowledge. Any world knowledge which does not directly specify the dynamics of communication can be considered separate from pragmatic knowledge 'that'. World knowledge can, of course, affect acquisition of pragmatic knowledge 'that' and the functioning of the pragmatic knowledge 'how', by providing input for these processes. Thus, knowing that humans interact for a purpose can be considered as one of the most basic types of pragmatic knowledge (see further below). Communication is defined as purposeful, intention-driven behaviour (Leech, 1983, Levinson, 1983).

Similarly, one can identify social, cultural and contextual knowledge which does not directly concern communication and can therefore be considered separate from, and at the same time interacting with, pragmatic knowledge. Such socio-cultural knowledge as 'a status difference may exist between adults and children, men and women or employer-employee' can be considered separate from such pragmatic knowledge as 'in adult–child, man–woman or employer–employee interaction certain conversational principles apply'. Similarly, knowledge of the defining characteristics of contexts (e.g. what defines a formal or an informal situation) can be considered distinct from knowledge of what constitutes appropriate communication in the specific contexts. The socio-cultural and contextual knowledge components essentially interact with pragmatic knowledge by feeding into the acquisition process and into the functioning of the procedural knowing 'how'. Knowing how to interact appropriately in specific societies/cultures and contexts presupposes knowledge of their defining characteristics. But such socio-cultural and contextual knowledge does not necessarily imply that this knowledge feeds into communication. One's ability to criticize one's own communicative behaviour after it has occurred illustrates that we can have knowledge which is not always functioning in communication. A link between these types of knowledge and pragmatic knowledge may not be made. On the other hand, pragmatic knowledge implies socio-cultural and contextual knowledge. Within this conceptualization, problems with socio-cultural, contextual and world knowledge can account for problems with pragmatic knowledge or with its mobilization (see further below). While this kind of demarcation between 'different types of knowledge' is essentially artificial, so interwoven is human functioning, it nevertheless serves a purpose of focusing one's attention on possible underlying causes or motivations for problematic communicative manifestations. It draws one's attention to the fact that communicative problems need not stem from lack of pragmatic knowledge or from problems with the 'knowing how'.

One further point needs to be considered. Is pragmatic 'knowing how', that is the knowledge which informs the selection and combination of knowledge for the purpose of communication, somehow different from some more general cognitive processing of knowledge? While we do not know the answer, it would appear that the personal needs and communicative purpose which motivate the pragmatic knowing 'how' impose restrictions upon how the different types of knowledge 'that' are to be combined.

Accumulation and linking of knowledge for one's own purposes can be idiosyncratic, unconcerned with socio-cultural and contextual norms or with the communicability or processability of the connections. Nor is one confined by what is possible in the world. This is not to suggest that the communicative purpose may not be fictional or imaginary but to suggest that communication is based on shared reality which communicators need to recognize (Levinson, 1983). Thus, pragmatic knowing 'how' is driven by communicative purpose and intention and the notion of mutual knowledge, thus differentiating it from a more general linking of ideas without the purpose of communication. The notions of interior and exterior discourse were discussed briefly in Chapter 1. It can be assumed that part of one's pragmatic knowing 'that' is knowing that a difference exists between interior and exterior discourse. It is also part of one's pragmatic knowing 'how' to make this distinction in communication. There may be some influences, such as psychiatric illness, which may render one unable to make this distinction or which may block one's ability to demonstrate that one knows this distinction. It may of course also be a possibility that the types of internal connections made by the mentally ill are somehow different from those made by 'normal' individuals.

ASPECTS OF THE PRAGMATIC 'KNOWING THAT'

An attempt will now be made to outline what pragmatic knowing 'that' entails: what one needs to know about communication to have a chance of functioning appropriately. This discussion is by no means exhaustive but simply provides a framework for conceptualizing pragmatic knowledge. The pragmatic knowing 'that' can be thought to consist of basic knowledge about communication and of knowledge which is specific to particular cultures and situations. The general aspects of pragmatic knowledge, on the other hand, are crucial for communication to occur at all. The general aspects of pragmatic knowing 'that' include the knowledge that

– one has a choice of communicating or not communicating with others;

- communication is co-operative, intention-driven be-haviour (speech act knowledge);
- communication is based on mutual knowledge; one needs to presuppose what the other person knows;
- one's communicative contribution needs to be relevant to the assumed shared topic;
- an expression can serve multiple communicative purposes;
- meanings can be negotiated in communication;
- there are expectations and consequences attached to communicative behaviour;
- intention can be expressed and interpreted directly or indirectly;
- items of information can be and need to be integrated with one another prior to being shared in communication;
- meanings can be shared via different signalling systems and modalities;
- when encountering a communication problem adaptation/ communication strategies can be used;
- exchanges of initiation and response take place in a variety of patterns and on a reciprocal basis;
- in order for communication to progress responses need to also function as initiations or have the possibility of doing so;
- one's own communicative behaviour has an effect on the mental state of others, potentially affecting their behaviour;
- one's own communicative behaviour has an effect on one's own being;
- different contexts and situations have different com-municative conventions associated with them;
- communicative behaviour can be appropriate or inappropriate;
- communicative behaviour can be judged appropriate or inappropriate in relation to contextual factors such as the status, age, sex, cultural origin or outlook of the participants, the setting and the discourse type;
- communicative behaviour can be judged successful or unsuccessful by oneself or others;
- the responsibility for successful communication may not be shared by the participants but ideally ought to be;
- one can attempt to clarify unclear messages and repair communication breakdown;

- the progress and interpretation of interaction can be regulated metacommunicatively;
- a consensus exists regarding what is salient in the world for communicative purposes;
- meanings expressed in communication can have personal significance for oneself and others;
- in communication one takes the other person's knowledge, interest and feelings into account, if one chooses;
- one can intentionally or unintentionally violate communicative principles;
- one can communicate about 'real' and imaginary objects, events and concepts;
- one can express one's opinion if one chooses and if the context permits.

While this representation of basic pragmatic knowledge is non-exhaustive, it serves the purpose of drawing attention to some of the possible deficits underlying 'odd', 'abnormal' or 'disordered' communicative manifestations.

Specific aspects of the pragmatic 'knowing that' reflecting socio-cultural and contextual influences can be identified in addition to the more general ones above. The specific aspects of pragmatic knowledge 'that' include the knowledge that

- a social rule forbids one to communicate in certain specific situations (e.g. women in certain cultures; in court; in church; in the theatre);
- a social rule requires one to communicate in certain situations (e.g. chatting at a party);
- one can use silence to make a specific point (e.g. be rude or unco-operative);
- a specific situation and/or communicative purpose may call for truthful or untruthful, informative or uninformative, brief or lengthy or ambiguous or unambiguous contributions;
- metacommunicative statements may need to be used for ascertaining the level of mutual knowledge;
- certain types of metacommunicative statement are likely to have certain effects;
- in a specific situation the expression used can serve specific purposes.

As these examples illustrate the specific knowledge 'that' reflects the application of the general knowledge 'that' in specific situations. It involves knowing that specific communicative situations call for detailed knowledge of what is socially, culturally and contextually appropriate and why. It is not sufficient to know that intention can be expressed or interpreted directly or indirectly or to know that 'shut up' is regarded as impolite; one must know that using this expression carries certain implications. However, in the early stages of communicative development one's specific pragmatic knowledge 'that' is unlikely to be very detailed. This is something which seems likely to become more sophisticated as life experiences increase.

Similar general accounts of the functioning of the pragmatic knowledge 'how' cannot be provided, since each instance of communication necessitates a specific integration of knowledge.

INFLUENCES BEARING UPON THE PRAGMATIC COMPONENT

Having discussed much of the literature on 'semantic-pragmatic disorder' and having explored the notion of a pragmatic component of communicative competence, it is now possible to examine communicative problems in more detail. Such problems are identified on the part of the client or others on the basis of behaviour or reception that appears unsuccessful, unusual, disturbing etc. (Chapter 4). On the basis of such subjective evaluations by clinicians and others individuals are labelled as 'semantic-pragmatic disordered'. A problem arises when the same communicative behaviours have different underlying motivations. The use of an all-embracing term, such as 'semantic-pragmatic disorder' may suggest homogeneity when we are almost certainly dealing with heterogeneous populations. Treatment based on such misconception is not likely to focus on the most appropriate aspects of the person's difficulty. The implications for research are also far-reaching. We propose a way of conceptualizing communication problems which takes these observations into account.

We can assume that communication is motivated by some

such pragmatic component as described above. That is to say that to exhibit appropriate and successful communicative behaviours and to interpret the behaviour of others one requires both declarative and procedural pragmatic knowledge. We can further assume that certain influences bear upon the way in which this knowledge is acquired, retained or used in actual communicative performance and in pragmatic comprehension. Some of these influences are likely to constrain the functioning of the pragmatic component.

Such constraining influences can be divided into those arising from the environment and those which exist within the client. The following serve as examples of such influences.

1. Environmental influences
    (a) Lack of input or disturbing input (e.g. different educational, social and cultural experiences from the person observing the behaviours; psychotic parent);
    (b) Lack of supportive or stimulating relationships; limited opportunity for high-quality interaction or limited contact with peer group;
    (c) Family tension, cruelty or abuse;
    (d) Inhibiting behaviour on the part of communicative partner in specific situations (e.g. domineering attitude; low expectation; inattention);
    (e) Restricting activities (e.g. picture naming; object sorting);
    (f) Unfamiliar, uninteresting or conceptually complex topics (e.g. cannot contribute to debate on astrophysics);
    (g) Intimidating communicative situation (e.g. courtroom; large group).
2. Within-client influences
    (h) Motor constraints (e.g. lack of ability to make oneself audible or intelligible; paralysis of the musculature involved in smiling;)
    (i) Inability to process with sufficient speed (e.g. a second language learner or a person with learning difficulties cannot keep up with rapid flow of conversation);

(j) Lack of confidence in one's ability to put the po-
     tential into actual use;
(k) Anxiety;
(l) Lack of interest and motivation, sometimes arising
     from (d) above;
(m) Noncommunicative personality (e.g. the recluse);
(n) Misperception of one's role in communication
     (e.g. not supposed to initiate; dominant partner
     at all times);
(o) Linguistic disability other than semantic (below);
(p) Psychiatric illness (e.g. those suffering from schizo-
     phrenia exhibit communication problems).

It is fairly easy to see that unsuccessful communicative
behaviours can reflect some of the factors above. Support
for some of these can be found in the research literature
(e.g. Brown, 1989; Schwartz, 1982; Yule and Rutter, 1987),
others are speculative, based on clinical observation and
experience.

There are factors which similarly affect communicative
behaviour but are more difficult to separate from the internal functioning of the pragmatic component. These
influencing factors include:

(q) Semantic deficit;
(r) Cognitive deficit;
(s) Learning deficit;
(t) 'Attention deficit';
(u) Neurological/biochemical deficit (genetic or acquired).

These are particularly difficult to disentangle because of
their interdependence on one another and the closeness
of their interrelatedness with the pragmatic component. It
seems likely that the internal functioning of the pragmatic
component is largely dependent on factors such as selective
attention, concept formation, vocabulary, memory and the
ability to interrelate pieces of information.

As with production, comprehension can also be influenced by factors such as those discussed above. Exceptions
would be factors (d), (e), (h), and (n). While the inclusions
and exclusions are largely self-explanatory, factor (i) needs
further comment. It is not uncommon to encounter clients

who do poorly in tests of sentence comprehension but whose performance can be improved by allowing them sufficient processing time and by providing additional prosodic cues. It is thus not surprising that the real-life demands of semantic and syntactic comprehension plus pragmatic integration frequently defeat such people, but what is encouraging is that real-life function benefits noticeably when clients are provided with assistance of the type just mentioned.

Factors such as the ones outlined above can be assumed to influence the functioning of the pragmatic component. This influence is reflected in inappropriate communicative behaviours. These factors and different combinations of them may affect the pragmatic component in the following ways.

1. The acquisition of pragmatic knowledge 'that' and/or 'how' is affected.
2. The retention of pragmatic knowledge 'that' and/or 'how' is affected.
3. The internal functioning of the pragmatic knowledge 'how' is affected; i.e. the way in which knowledge is selected and combined in communicatively appropriate ways.
4. The mobilization of the pragmatic component is affected.

1, 2 and 3 refer to a situation in which the internal functioning of the pragmatic component is being affected, while in the case of 4 only the external functioning suffers. In the latter case, some influences are blocking the appropriate external functioning of an intact pragmatic component. In other words, it is only the mobilization of the pragmatic knowledge which is constrained.

It can be suggested that negative influences which bear upon an individual's pragmatic behaviour rather than on the underlying pragmatic component might begin to affect the underlying knowledge, in certain circumstances. These are likely to include factors such as repeated opportunity for the influence to operate, the personal significance of the prevented behaviour and the specific combinations of influences which bear upon the pragmatic component at any one time. To take an example, let us imagine a person who knows that one is expected to make a verbal contribution in formal meetings ('pragmatic knowing that') and also knows what constitutes an appropriate contribution at any specific point in the meeting ('pragmatic knowing how'). Let us also assume that this person has a fear of speaking in front of other people and thus more often than not fails to make a contribution. Accordingly, the person's pragmatic knowledge is intact and it is the mobilization of this knowledge which is prevented by the personal fear. The pragmatic 'being able' is overridden by the person 'feeling unable'. Let us further assume that this person goes to many meetings, and thus not making an expected contribution occurs a great deal, reinforcing the fear component and the feelings of inadequacy. As a consequence, the person may become unsure when it is appropriate to make a contribution and how one should be made: the pragmatic 'knowing how' may become fuzzy. It is difficult to imagine in relation to this example that the actual 'pragmatic knowing that' could become affected but in the case of prolonged institutionalization of patients their once adequate pragmatic knowledge 'that' might well become fuzzy, or even forgotten.

This characterization of deterioration of the pragmatic component questions the validity of approaches which seem to consider the notion of pragmatic disturbance a matter of either–or. The term 'semantic-pragmatic disorder' implies a dichotomous distinction 'disordered' or 'not disordered' while those categorized as 'disordered' are likely to exhibit variation in the extent and degree of their communicative functioning, depending on specific contexts. The terms 'pragmatic disturbance' and 'pragmatic deficit' are preferable, reflecting the indeterminate and fluid nature of pragmatic functioning. They capture the problematic nature of the notion of appropriacy in communication (Chapter 6). They also shift the responsibility for successful communication from the client's shoulders to the 'broader shoulders' of the dynamics of the whole communication process.

Most of the influences bearing upon the pragmatic component can affect both its internal and external functioning. It is not difficult to see that all of the influences can constrain the acquisition of pragmatic knowledge, some, however, seeming more obviously damaging than others. They all have potential for preventing a child from experiencing the type of interaction which may be necessary for the acquisition of pragmatic knowledge. A child who is perceived as strange may not be talked to or played with, thus losing opportunities to receive the necessary input and gain confidence in communication. Such a child may lose not only interactive opportunities but also the facilitative effects of these on interior discourse. Thoughts are normally elaborated and consolidated in conjunction with other people, a process which is not available to the social isolate. Some of these influences which can directly affect input (e.g. lack of input, disturbing input, lack of supporting or stimulating relationships) are environmental. In addition, within-client influences which are either crucial for the pragmatic component to function at all (e.g. semantic, cognitive, and neurological deficits) or influences which affect the client's learning process (e.g. inability to process with sufficient speed; childhood psychiatric illness; linguistic disability; 'attention deficit'; non-communicative personality; anxiety; lack of confidence) can have an effect on acquisition. There are also influences which may interfere with the pragmatic acquisition process less directly. These include motor constraints, client's misperception of their role in communication, intimidating communicative situation and restricting activities.

PRAGMATIC KNOWLEDGE AND SEVERITY OF DISTURBANCE

The conceptualization of pragmatic disturbance presented here enables one to explore how one might determine the degree of severity. The severity of pragmatic problems can be approached from different points of view, which may suggest different severity ratings.

1. from the point of view of the client's personal and communicative needs;
2. from the point of view of those interacting with the client;
3. from the point of view of remediability;

4. from the point of view of the functioning of the pragmatic component.

Let us consider each of these briefly.

1. Having problems with the internal or external functioning of the pragmatic component can compromise the client's personal and communicative needs. As was suggested in Chapter 3 (Section 'Communication strategies'), compromising one's personal goals can have a more detrimental effect on one as a communicator, and as a human being, than when compromising one's communicative goals. Personal goals can be perceived as the motivating force for communication to occur at all.

2. What one needs to bear in mind is that most judgements concerning severity of pragmatic disturbance tend to be based on the initial judgement of what one as an observer finds disturbing (Chapter 4). Some such conceptual framework as outlined here enables one to move from these initial hypotheses into more 'objective' (Chapter 2) considerations of the nature and severity of the disturbance.

3. Whether or not anything can be done to remedy pragmatic problems may depend upon which aspect of the pragmatic component is being affected and by which influences. For instance, influences reflecting neurological or cognitive deficits are likely to be more difficult to remediate than influences stemming from the environment or from such within-client influences as anxiety or lack of confidence. The environmental influences, being 'outside the client', can be thought of as potentially less detrimental for the pragmatic component, which is still 'potentially more able'; the acquisition process is being affected by influences which can potentially be addressed. Those influences within the client which are crucial for the acquisition of pragmatic knowledge and for the functioning of the pragmatic component render the pragmatic component, and therefore the person, 'potentially less able'. Remediation is likely to be more problematic and time consuming in the latter case.

4. When the pragmatic component is internally affected by the influences, the pragmatic component can be said to be 'potentially less able'. When the influences have an

effect on the mobilization of intact pragmatic knowledge rather than on its internal functioning, the pragmatic component can be said to be 'potentially more able'. The influences which initially affect only the mobilization can, however, as indicated above, gradually penetrate the pragmatic component.

The potential destructiveness of the influences on the functioning of the pragmatic component can be further refined. Having effect on the acquisition of 'the knowing that' can be said to be more detrimental for the pragmatic component than having effect on the acquisition of 'the knowing how'. This is because 'the knowing that' component feeds into (i.e. provides input for) 'the knowing how' (see section above). As has been discussed above, 'the knowing that' constitutes the store of pragmatic knowledge from which 'the knowing how' selects and combines in communicatively appropriate ways.

Furthermore, 'the knowing that' can be divided into aspects of knowledge which are more or less crucial for the functioning of the pragmatic component. 'Knowing that meanings can be shared with others'; 'knowing that one has choices'; 'knowing that communicative actions produce reactions'; 'knowing that one needs to be appropriate'; 'knowing that one can make statements, ask questions, insult, joke etc.'; 'knowing that one ought not to mention the war to grandad' signify general and more specific types of pragmatic knowledge. One requires the most general type of pragmatic knowledge to have a chance of functioning at all and the more specific types to have a chance of functioning appropriately in specific situations.

This severity criterion could conflict with criterion number 1 above, concerning clients' personal and communicative needs. Such influences as anxiety or no opportunity to communicate which may only block the functioning of otherwise intact pragmatic knowledge can, however, seriously compromise one's functioning as a communicator.

SEMANTIC-PRAGMATIC DISORDER?

If we accept that one's pragmatic behaviour results from the interaction of many underlying motivations and evolves and unfolds within the dynamics of communication then it is not difficult to appreciate that heterogeneity is a more likely characteristic of populations exhibiting communication problems than homogeneity. Homogeneity is likely to be merely a surface phenomenon, reflecting similarity in actual communicative behaviours. In clinical contexts, where remediation is targeted at underlying causes, it is crucial to recognize the heterogeneous nature of these causes and their different potential effects on underlying pragmatic knowledge. All-embracing terms, such as 'semantic-pragmatic disorder' can therefore be more misleading than helpful. It may be more helpful to consider odd, inappropriate etc. communicative behaviours or absence of expected behaviours as reflecting pragmatic disturbance either in the internal functioning of the pragmatic component or its external mobilization. Some of this disturbance may reflect a deficit in the pragmatic knowledge component. Therefore, it may be more useful in the clinical context to describe the nature of the disturbance and to speculate on the potential underlying causes rather than simply label on the basis of behavioural manifestations.

Where does this leave the notion of 'semantic-pragmatic disorder'? The current conceptualization highlights three major problems with the notion of 'disorder' in the context of pragmatic problems. Within the medical model, disorder implies that something specifiable is at fault. In relation to pragmatics, it implies that something is at fault that is specific to one's pragmatic functioning. Appropriate communication does not originate from any one specific source; it evolves and unfolds as a result of a complex integration of personal abilities, feelings and contextual influences. As such, one cannot pinpoint precisely where apparent communicative inappropriacy stems from. All that one can say is that something is influencing the underlying pragmatic component which manifests itself in communication problems. This does not imply that we cannot specify many of the factors which contribute to the misfunctioning of the pragmatic component but rather that there may not be any one aspect of human functioning which is responsible for 'pragmatics'.

Secondly, the notion of 'disorder' places responsibility for adequate acquisition of pragmatic knowledge and appropriate communicative functioning with the client. Undoubtedly, some communication problems do originate from the client. But, as has been outlined above, inappropriate communicative behaviours are likely to result from a combination of within- and outside-client factors. Because of the complex interrelatedness of these factors it may be impossible to distinguish between the two types. Indeed, it is quite unlikely that one's pragmatic problems would solely reflect one type or the other. Furthermore, those influencing factors which exist within a client do not necessarily reflect something being 'wrong' with one's pragmatic ability; one may not be able or feel able to mobilize existing knowledge. Because of the difficulty in determining whether the client is at 'fault' or not, and if he/she is, for what reason, it may be wiser to avoid such potentially damaging labels as 'disordered' or 'deviant'.

The third point is closely related to the previous one. A dictionary definition of the term 'disorder' reminds one of its medical origin: 'an upset of health; ailment; a deviation from the normal system or order' (The New Collins Concise English Dictionary, 1982). It is difficult to see how pragmatic problems constitute a health problem. Some pragmatic problems can indeed stem from an underlying medical 'ailment' but obviously not all. Similar problems arise with the second part of this definition. What might constitute 'the normal pragmatic system'? Could the notion of a pragmatic system parallel the notion of a linguistic system? A person's pragmatic component, while likely to consist of universal and culturally based features, is an ultimate reflection of a person's life experiences and personal needs. It is also a reflection of the person's significant others. Because of this, no ultimate norm can exist. Deviations from universally and culturally based norms can be identified, yet on a much more subjective basis than when identifying, let us say, problems with grammatical structures of specific languages. As indicated above, pragmatic problems are not 'either-or' entities but hinge upon the notion of degree; the notion of 'disorder', on the other hand, minimizes the notion of continuum and consequently the possibility of gradual deterioration of the pragmatic knowledge component.

Turning to the 'semantic-pragmatic' part of the term

'semantic-pragmatic disorder' several observations can be made. Firstly, having the terms 'semantic' and 'pragmatic' so closely interlinked in this context can have several implications:

1. One's semantic and pragmatic functioning are so interwoven that they cannot be separated. This does not appear a likely interpretation in that some aspects of one's communicative functioning are clearly based on 'pragmatic knowledge' only (e.g. 'knowing that one has choices'; 'knowing that one can be polite or impolite') and some others on 'semantic knowledge' only (e.g. 'knowing the meaning of a specific word'). Some aspects of one's pragmatic functioning are, however, dependent on semantic functioning (e.g. cannot actually request specific information without access to the meanings of individual words).

2. Semantic problems entail pragmatic problems. At first sight it may appear that if one has semantic problems it might be hard to escape pragmatic failure. Productively, one's options would be limited, while receptively, one would fail to respond appropriately to utterances containing unfamiliar words. However, whether or not inappropriate pragmatic behaviour occurs will depend on whether the mobilization of intact pragmatic knowledge is blocked by semantic deficit or whether the semantic deficit has affected the pragmatic knowledge itself. In the former instance, the use of communication strategies could prevent the occurrence of pragmatically inappropriate behaviour (Chapter 3). For instance, a person might apologize for not knowing the polite expression for making a request. In the latter instance, our perception of the influence of semantic knowledge upon pragmatic knowledge is less clear. This is an area which urgently requires investigation (but see Lucas, 1983).

3. Pragmatic problems entail semantic problems. In general this is not the case. Having problems with the functioning of the pragmatic component does not interfere with the functioning of the semantic component. Pragmatic problems can, however, influence the acquisition of semantic knowledge. Lack of input for semantic

acquisitions could result from failure to interact satisfactorily with others. Some types of pragmatic problem,
however, would not affect the acquisition of concepts
and meaning. For instance, the inability to maintain
topics does not necessarily reduce input because other
people tend to compensate.

On the basis of this brief exploration it appears that the
concepts 'semantic' and 'pragmatic' are not as closely interlinked as the term 'semantic-pragmatic disorder' might
suggest. Following our current conceptualization of pragmatic disturbance, the term 'semantic' can be envisaged
as reflecting one of the influences bearing upon the pragmatic component. Until it can be proven that semantic
and pragmatic functioning are somehow more intrinsically
interwoven than, let us say, other linguistic, cognitive or
emotional aspects of one's being, semantic aspects of one's
communicative component need not be given additional
emphasis in the context of pragmatic disturbance. This is
in line with the importance we wish to place on the recognition of the varied nature of potential underlying causes
of communication problems which broad-cover terms fail to
address. This use of 'semantic' in conjunction with 'pragmatic' by clinicians, however, is motivated by a consistent
observation that children who demonstrate pragmatic difficulties frequently fail to 'understand' situations, needs,
messages and implications. In these circumstances, the
clinician's training suggests investigation of semantic comprehension. Sure enough, semantic problems do surface
(Rapin and Allen, 1987). Nevertheless, they do not necessarily account for the pragmatic nature of the failures. For
instance, lack of semantic specificity hardly accounts for
a failure to integrate literal meaning with situational requirements, neither can limitations of vocabulary account
for inability to draw together information so as to derive
coherent and meaningful ideas (Frith, 1989). In order to
make progress in understanding the serious pragmatic
difficulties of autistic children or the less severe but none-
theless incapacitating difficulties of those labelled 'semantic-
pragmatic disordered' it will be necessary to explore in
detail the various aspects of pragmatic knowledge. The

current conceptualization based on Faerch and Kasper (1984) provides a starting point for such an exploration. However, a great deal of thinking remains to be done.

Relevant to this discussion is the notion of 'specific pragmatic disorder'. Following the medical model, it is customary in clinical professions to identify specific under- lying causes for 'abnormal' manifestations. In relation to 'semantic-pragmatic disorders' attempts have been made at identifying groups of individuals whose communication problems appear to stem from specific disturbance to their pragmatic functioning. Such specific disturbance could be neurologically based (Bayles and Boone, 1982; Code, 1987; Bryan, 1988). If neurological impairment can be considered as the major contributing factor for the dysfunctioning of the pragmatic component, the problem could be termed 'specific'. Such identification would rest upon elimination of other possible causes. Given the difficulty of deter- mining exact causes of communication problems and of determining the relative weight of the various contributing factors, two fundamental points need to be kept in mind. To ignore neurological impairment which alters the indi- vidual's ability in some fundamental way (rendering them 'less pragmatically able'; see above) reduces options for appropriate remedial and compensatory strategies. On the other hand, giving undue weight to one of many factors which bear upon the individual's performance obscures one's view of the other contributing factors, thereby dis- torting one's conceptualization of the difficulty. The reason why a more integrative approach is recommended is that it contributes towards a more realistic appraisal of the person's communicative potential. It also enables one to monitor conditions which contribute to the perpetuation or amelioration of that person's difficulties.

It is also useful to recognize at this point that consider- ing language difficulties as being closely interlinked with pragmatic disturbance may also focus one's attention un- duly on one relationship at the cost of ignoring other equally valid associations. As is apparent in the literature review above, pragmatic problems have been considered as an aspect of a more general notion of language disability. This perception rests upon the notion that pragmatics is a level of language, in line with the phonological, syntactic, semantic, and possibly, discourse levels. This is what Craig (1983, 102) refers to as the 'narrow interpretation of pragmatic theory', pragmatics being 'conceptualized simply as another set of language skills' emphasizing 'use' rather than the structural properties of language. In contrast, pragmatics can be considered within a wider perspective in which all communicative functioning, be it linguistic or non-verbal, is integrated within an overriding pragmatic framework and is motivated by one's attempt to make sense of the world (Searle, 1969, Halliday, 1975, Craig, 1983). 'Much of the clinical promise of pragmatics' (Craig, 1983, 102) is ignored when treatment design is influenced only by the narrow view. Similarly, the narrow view can lead to diagnosis which ignores the common thread which underlies all communication by focusing solely on the use of language.

PRAGMATIC CONTINUUM

It is useful to relate the notions of 'knowing that' and 'how' to the communication pathology context. Different severities of communication disorders can be related to the different aspects of the pragmatic component. Those children who appear not to be communicating at all or only very minimally can be said to have problems with the acquisition of the very general features of the knowing 'that'. Candidates for this could be severe cases of childhood autism (Bishop and Rosenbloom, 1987). Less severe cases of autism and Asperger's Syndrome (Wing, 1988) could reflect problems with less general aspects of the knowing 'that' and the knowledge of how to select and combine these into appropriate manifestations. The 'semantic-pragmatic disorder or syndrome' in children (Rapin and Allen, 1983; Bishop and Rosenbloom, 1987) being primarily characterized by inappropriate communicative behaviours can be assumed to reflect problems in the selection and integration of the different types of declarative knowledge 'that'. This problem may stem from the knowledge of 'how' not being fully acquired in the first instance or if acquired not appropriately functioning. The common thread between the three is the problem in the functioning of the pragmatic component; the differences lie in which aspects of this knowledge have failed to be acquired, retained or mobilized. The three syndromes can be said to constitute a pragmatic deficit, reflecting different degrees of severity. They can be regarded as points on a 'pragmatic continuum' (Wing, 1988, Bishop, 1989 in the literature review above).

ISSUE OF DIAGNOSIS

As a profession accustomed to making confident diagnoses of speech and language disorder, speech pathologists have experienced some dismay on being confronted with a new category of a disorder which is so unclear. Clinically, the conceptualization described in this chapter implies that remedial focus shifts away from accurate diagnosis leading to appropriate treatment. People whose communicative behaviours are perceived as odd will be looked at in relation to a number of specific considerations rather than being given a simplistic label which sheds little light on the true nature of the problem. This is not to minimize the value of diagnosing. Families and clients can be assisted by the confirmation of the presence or absence of 'real' obstacles to progress. Teachers and colleagues may interact more sympathetically with people who are seen as having bona fide disabilities than with those who are perceived as uncomfortable conversational partners. The client's self-esteem can also be affected by diagnosis. Students and clinicians are assisted in devising suitable treatment programmes when their diagnosis is correct. Research is facilitated by accurate diagnosis, providing well-defined subject populations. However, the concept of pragmatic disturbance is likely to take some time to become sufficiently stable for there to be terminological and procedural agreement between the professions concerned with its diagnosis. Meanwhile, well-informed exploration and description of communicative events and their potential motivations might prove less misleading and more informative than premature diagnosis. Rapin and Allen (1983) lamented that in the case of one young man known to them, 'again and again those who did not understand the neurological basis of his problem viewed him as psychotic' (p. 176). A detailed description of this man's problems suggested a 'semantic-pragmatic syndrome without autism'.

A further concern in diagnosis involves the manipulation of terms for administrative purposes. The families of people with unusual communication difficulties report a feeling of vulnerability due to the rulings of insurance companies or administrative bodies that funding, placements and facilities can be made available in the event of certain diagnoses rather than others. Even 'recovery' has been known to coincide with the exhaustion of funds for treatment. A more satisfactory procedure now widely adopted is for professionals, client and family to construct descriptive reports, with possible diagnoses forming part of such reports. In this way a picture of the strengths and needs of the client emerges together with some indication of treatable conditions and projected outcomes.

SUMMARY

What the current conceptualization suggests is that 'odd' communicative behaviours, describable in terms of categories in clinical pragmatic protocols (Chapter 6), are not necessarily indicative of something being 'wrong' with the underlying pragmatic component. Nor do such behaviours and categorizations (necessarily) suggest a 'semantic-pragmatic disorder'. What has been suggested here is a way of conceptualizing the relationship between actual behaviour and underlying pragmatic knowledge. This conceptualization is based on influences bearing upon the functioning of the pragmatic component and their potentially differential effects on the pragmatic potential for 'being able'. It is recognized that 'being potentially able', that is having an intact pragmatic component, does not imply that one 'actually does'. It also acknowledges the importance of not only 'being able' but also the 'feeling able' and 'being allowed to be able' aspects in communication. It is also appreciated that pragmatic problems can be fairly indeterminate in nature, as are notions of communicative appropriacy and acceptability; therefore the notion of degrees of pragmatic disturbance is relevant (Bishop and Rosenbloom, 1987). This also ties up with the possibility of the pragmatic component becoming gradually affected by various types of influences some of which are susceptible to intervention. Incorporating the possibility that others can influence the pragmatic knowledge of the client and the way in which this knowledge becomes mobilized, shares the responsibility for communicative success and failure between interactants. It is reasonable to suppose that communication problems can manifest solely because of environmental influences or because these influences may compound with within-client influences to exaggerate the pragmatic problem.

Clinically this conceptualization, which allows for competence without performance and for variability of performance in different circumstances, provides a framework for describing problems and determining their severity. Where treatment is concerned the focus is shifted from surface behaviour to underlying motivation and knowledge. The importance of integrating and co-ordinating knowledge and skills is acknowledged, as is the mutual responsibility of all participants in interaction. As a result methods which take the client's environment into consideration and which strike a balance between behaviour-change and knowledge-change are recommended. More specific hypothetical recommendation for assessment and remediation can also be made. It can be suggested that assessment might determine whether the acquisition, retention, the internal functioning and/or the mobilization of the pragmatic component is affected and for what reasons. Tasks could be designed to investigate whether and which aspects of the 'knowing that' or the 'knowing how' are being affected.

Chapter 6

Pragmatic assessment

Pragmatic assessment can be regarded as fundamental to all other assessments in speech-language remediation, because it is how a client uses language, or an alternative system, to think, learn and communicate that determines whether or not there is a need for intervention. Later, when it has been discovered what the client's primary requirements are, a detailed analysis of the component parts of communicative ability may be necessary. Without some form of pragmatic assessment it is not possible to prioritize the steps by which client and clinician together will attempt to manage a communicative problem. Skilled clinicians have always undertaken this prioritizing exercise, whether or not they have employed the term 'pragmatics' to do so. Our suggestion is that the most realistic goals for intervention are those which emphasize the personal usefulness of alterations in attitude, behaviour, knowledge or skill, which the clinician and the client together are able to bring about.

Assessment of the adequacy of the client's communicative performance has traditionally therefore been part of the clinical procedure. On the basis of this initial assessment hypotheses concerning the client's communicative abilities are made. The difficulty of assessing underlying ability on the basis of performance can become forgotten in the clinical situation. It can be too readily assumed that therapy must be targeted at disability and that inadequate performance therefore indicates disability on which the therapist can get to work; whereas therapy which is targeted at mobilizing existing abilities which have been concealed by poor performance may be equally legitimate.

Other than for the researcher, assessment is undertaken

with therapy in mind involving two major considerations: firstly, the need for the client and the family to experience early success and secondly, the relative destructiveness to communication of particular shortcomings. Early success can be provided by identifying skills toward which the client feels motivated. Once the client has experienced success, treatment goals can be based on more detailed and principled assessments designed to reveal those behaviours which render the client communicatively inadequate. (For instance, lack of some phonological contrasts is likely to affect intelligibility more than lack of others; Chapter 4.)

In order to arrive at realistic treatment goals, clinicians usually conduct assessments in a certain sequence. The first step is to gain an informal impression of the client as a communicator by piecing together any available information obtained in the process of getting to know the client. The next step is to discover whether the client is eager for help or whether it is family or others who desire intervention. How clients perceive themselves in relation to speech therapy will affect their motivation and this in turn exerts a powerful influence on the outcome of therapy. In parallel with this step, assessment involves determining whether there is a need to refer clients for specialist attention of other kinds (e.g. medical). The third stage of assessment concerns more formal appraisal of linguistic and pragmatic skills. Since linguistic functioning occurs within pragmatic context, we suggest that pragmatic assessment should underpin linguistic assessment.

Detailed pragmatic assessment is a skilled professional undertaking, belying the apparent simplicity of clinicians' activities with clients, and no anxiety need be felt if the outcome of thorough assessment indicates a need for 'relaxed' therapy. The professional value of pragmatic assessment might however be challenged in the absence of adequate normative developmental data, which potentially renders such assessments less attractive because of the pressures of financial accountability. However, accountability to clients themselves is well served by pragmatic assessment even in the absence of adequate normative data, since it is able to reveal generally accepted areas of strength and need in the client (Chapter 10).

One of the primary goals in carrying out linguistic as-sessment has been the identification of disorder and dis-ability (Crystal, Fletcher and Garman, 1976, Grunwell, 1985, Stoel-Gammon and Dunn, 1985). The objective of this identification is to enable one to estimate prognosis and to make general and specific recommendations for management and treatment. Assessment also enables clinicians to monitor progress, to give early warning of progressive conditions, to identify unsuitable placement, to reverse unnecessary (i.e. socially mediated) deterioration and to intervene in the correct area (e.g. by spending time talking with relatives rather than inappropriately coaching the client). In order to move towards these objectives it is necessary to obtain and analyse representative samples of the client's communicative behaviour and, where possible, to compare the analysis with normative data. Trying to fulfil these objectives in relation to specific linguistic prob-lems has proved difficult, but given the complex nature of pragmatic functioning and the resulting difficulty of determining what might constitute a pragmatic disorder (Chapter 5), the problems are compounded in the case of pragmatic assessment. Having examined some inherent dif-ficulties with the concept of 'pragmatic disorder' (Chapter 5), it nevertheless needs to be acknowledged that clients exist who have major problems with sharing meaning in com-munication and that an attempt needs to be made to assess and treat these people. The aim of this chapter is to draw attention to some of the potential pitfalls in pragmatic as-sessment and to collate information on existing methods. McTear and Conti-Ramsden (1989) have recently explored these issues in relation to types of pragmatic assessment and outlined some points for future consideration. These suggestions will be incorporated into the current discussion.

ISSUES IN SAMPLING

Methods of obtaining representative samples of a client's language or communicative behaviour and problems as-sociated with these methods have been acknowledged in the literature (e.g. Johnston, Weinrich and Johnson, 1984). Before we can begin to explore what might constitute a representative sample for pragmatic assessment and how one might go about obtaining one, it needs to be clarified what the term 'representative' entails. Gallagher (1983, 3) discusses three different senses of the term as used in the literature: she considers representative behaviour as 'comprehensive', as 'idealized' and as 'typical' behaviour. The term 'comprehensive' refers to a sample which, while being small enough to be manageable, is large enough to have the possibility of including the behaviours one wishes to examine. Comprehensiveness may not be difficult to achieve when dealing with phenomena of definable size such as adult target phonology but is likely to be an impossible aim when dealing with the complex integration of factors giving rise to pragmatic phenomena. Also, the scope and variability of appropriate pragmatic behaviour is such that by specifying target behaviours one unjustifiably restricts one's view of successful participation on the part of the client. For instance, expected responses to 'What's this?' might be 'Apple' or 'Eat it' whereas unexpected but equally legitimate responses could be 'Well, an apple of course' or 'Don't you know?' When discussing comprehensiveness of data samples, linguistic assessment protocols recommend certain sizes of samples (Crystal, Fletcher and Garman, 1976, Bloom and Lahey, 1978, Miller, 1981, Grunwell, 1985). For pragmatic assessment such recommendations cannot be provided. A rough guide as to whether a reasonable sample of a client's behaviour has been recorded can, however, be obtained by consulting those familiar with the client's communicative repertoire.

The second aspect of representativeness, that of idealized or optimal behaviour, concerns the danger of under- or over-estimating a client's abilities. Making sure that the best performance of which the client is capable has been observed maximizes the possibility of making a realistic assessment. As with comprehensiveness, the guidance of those who know the client best is valuable. One does not then ignore reports of better performance on better days, neither does one over-estimate on the basis of stereotyped or coached performance.

Similarly, typicality of performance can only be estimated by those who know the client well. Typical performance portrays the client's 'usual', 'habitual', 'most frequent' or 'daily' communicative performance. Gallagher's (1983) Pre-Assessment Questionnaire is designed to handle the issue of representativeness by gathering information about the client's communicative habits and potential in different contexts involving different partners, different purposes and different environments.

Variability is a further consideration in sampling. Within the medical model, variable performance is considered as one of the manifestations of pathology. However, when engaging in communicative behaviour, being able to vary one's performance appropriately is the very essence of pragmatic skill. This being the case, sampling should, if possible, capture the client's ability or inability to vary performance according to circumstances.

How to obtain representative samples for communicative assessment has been widely discussed. Miller (1981), for instance, provides detailed guidance for interacting with children in a manner likely to provide a representative spontaneous language sample. Our purpose here is not to repeat these guidelines, which if followed are likely to produce typical or even optimal samples of client's spontaneous pragmatic behaviour within one context, but to add two further suggestions.

Firstly, in order to obtain a typical and an optimal sample for assessment of linguistic skill, sampling in different communicative contexts is essential (Lund and Duchan, 1983, Muma, 1983, Prutting and Kirchner, 1983, Roth and Spekman, 1984a,b). Sampling in varying contexts for the purposes of pragmatic assessment is also recommended as a means of tapping a variety of pragmatic behaviours and skills and as a means of observing the client's ability to vary performance according to circumstances. This measure enhances representativeness.

Secondly, linguistic assessment is ideally based on spontaneous or free conversational samples in order to capture what a client is capable of doing when not being prompted, and therefore aided or restricted. Pragmatic assessment, being primarily interested in the client's ability to use knowledge in communication, requires a similar client-driven communicative sample. However, since 'pragmatics' involves integration of a great variety of knowledge and skills and since appropriateness is ultimately a speaker/ listener/ context-specific notion it may need to be accepted that one can never be sure how much of this knowledge and integration can be inferred on the basis of a spontaneous sample. The alternative of elicitation of data by use of specific tasks and tests poses a similar problem of interpretation, yet it offers the possibility of a more systematic and principled investigation of pragmatic potential. The way forward may be that of systematic and optimal narrowing of the focus of pragmatic assessment where only one or a few aspects of pragmatic functioning will be targeted at any one time. Such systematic narrowing of the focus calls for a hypothesis as to the nature of the pragmatic phenomenon. In Chapter 5, a hypothesis concerning the nature of the relationship between pragmatic skill and knowledge was put forward which may provide some impetus for construction of specific pragmatic tasks for specific purposes. In the narrowing of the focus, problems similar to those already identified by McTear and Conti-Ramsden (1989) in relation to pragmatic tests (e.g. Shulman, 1985) are likely to surface. Too much information might be lost. Therefore, a combination of spontaneous and elicited information is essential.

Pragmatic comprehension, that is the integration and evaluation of incoming information, presents a unique set of problems for assessment. Because of the unobservability of comprehension, be it semantic or pragmatic in nature, it can only be accessed impressionistically and/or by means of targeted probes. The challenge in assessment is to determine which probes target which specific aspects of comprehension. Again, a hypothesis concerning the nature of pragmatic comprehension is required in order to be able to construct specific comprehension tasks in a systematic manner. The hypothesis explored in Chapter 5 may prove useful in this endeavour.

ISSUES IN ANALYSIS AND INTERPRETATION

Once samples of data have been obtained for pragmatic assessment, the question of how to analyse the data arises (that is, if we are not dealing with tests). Analysis of data for pragmatic purposes presents many problems. Firstly, it is not clear what constitutes suitable pragmatic behaviour for analysis and assessment. This problem stems from a more basic difficulty of determining what constitutes pragmatic ability or disability, which in turn reflects a difficulty in determining what pragmatic knowledge and skill might entail (Chapter 5). Without attempting to interrelate the very basis of pragmatic problems with analysis and assessment one could carry out detailed and intricate analyses which might be incidental or even irrelevant for exploring the true nature of the problem. This is not to suggest that the current approaches to pragmatic assessment necessarily fail to capture behaviours that are 'pragmatic' in nature, but to emphasize the need for some systematic theory for exploring what pragmatic ability or disability means. It is within such a theory that one can then explore how to assess pragmatic problems. While recognizing that one can never be totally sure what one is assessing on the basis of communicative manifestations, a theoretically based exploration would at least generate hypotheses which could provide an impetus for further exploration. In line with the discussion of 'pragmatic disorder' in Chapter 5, assessment protocols based on the notions of different types of pragmatic knowledge and skill might provide a future direction. A method using the cognitive dimensions of selection and integration as diagnostic and assessment parameters in language disability is currently being investigated (Ottem, 1990, Bollingmo and Ottem, 1990), and is also likely to provide insight into assessment of pragmatic disturbance. This kind of exploration could also provide some clarification as to the boundaries of semantic and pragmatic problems (e.g. Landells, 1989).

A second major problem of pragmatic assessment concerns lack of normative data. The question of what constitutes developmentally normal pragmatic behaviour may prove to be an inappropriate one. Both cross-sectional and longitudinal studies of communicative development in children are emerging, yet generalizing from specific studies to 'a general child population' is particularly problematic in the pragmatic domain. This difficulty reflects the context-

specific nature of communication and the numerous influences which shape one's behaviour. When trying to
describe what constitutes 'normal' pragmatic behaviour,
one can more often than not think of situations where behaviours not falling within a 'normal' range could be deemed
appropriate and acceptable. Because of such indeterminacy,
what might prove to be more useful are explorations of
the boundaries of variability. A central aspect of pragmatic
ability is the ability to vary one's performance according to
circumstances and thus studies addressing the development of one's ability to vary and adapt might provide a
realistic angle for communicative development. For instance, children have been observed to use different communicative behaviours when interacting with peers as
compared with adults. If we simply know the differences
but not when and how children begin to identify the differences and act accordingly and if we do not study the
likely resultant variability in one's behaviour surfacing
in the developmental process, we have a very static view
of communicative development and ability. It has been
reported that children identified as 'pragmatically' disordered have problems with matching of behaviour with
context (e.g. Rapin and Allen, 1983, Prutting and Kirchner,
1983, Bishop and Adams, 1989). Knowledge of the developmental process of 'appropriate contextualization' would
thus prove useful.

The key issue when discussing shortage of information
concerning developmental norms for pragmatic behaviour
is the elusiveness of the notion of communicative appropriacy and inappropriacy. The judgement of appropriacy is
context-dependent and socio-culturally motivated. Appropriacy is ultimately a subjective experience on the part of
the observer, resting on one's life experiences, one's purpose for the observation, one's tolerance for 'the unusual'
and similar factors (Chapter 1). Yet, some concensus exists
between different individuals with regard to behaviours
being communicatively inappropriate in specific contexts.
Bishop and Adams (1989), for instance, found agreement
amongst three individual raters when identifying instances
of inappropriacy in conversations involving 'normally' developing children, language impaired children and children

diagnosed as 'semantically-pragmatically disordered'. Inappropriate utterances were deemed to be those that produced 'a sense of oddness and disruption of the normal conversational flow' (p. 242). Grammatical ill-formedness was discounted. Bishop and Adams also identified types of communicative indices which appeared to give rise to the sense of inappropriacy. These included a wide range of semantic, syntactic and pragmatic characteristics. The question of why raters find certain behaviours appropriate and not others needs also to be asked. Since inappropriacy is an observer-centred notion, it does not suffice to find that agreement exists. In order to explore the legitimacy of this agreement what are needed are explorations of why adult raters tend to perceive similar child behaviours as inappropriate. By asking this question, one can explore whether the reasons are based on adult conversational 'norms' and expectations and whether these are realistic in relation to child communication. The idea that one's view of communicative success and failure is influenced by the perspective one operates with, and that one's perspective may not be the only possible one, requires further thought (Leinonen and Smith, 1989, McTear and Conti-Ramsden, 1989). It is interesting to note that in the Bishop and Adams study, the 'independent raters' were the two authors and a speech therapist who was given three hours of training with examples of utterances which were agreed to be inappropriate by both authors. The notion of appropriacy/inappropriacy in discourse requires further study, which examines why observers identify communicative behaviours as appropriate/inappropriate.

One further point about the notion of appropriacy is its relationship to the notion of communication or compensatory strategy (Chapter 3). Inappropriacy implies behaviours which are undesirable and which thus become targets for change or elimination. Behaviours such as circumlocution, topic shift or style-switching, for instance, might render a piece of discourse inappropriate by rendering it stylistically awkward or inefficient. While from the point of view of the observer these behaviours may be judged inappropriate, from the point of view of the client they can be indices of active compensatory strategies developed to cope with one's communicative weaknesses. Indeed, from the client's point of view, such inappropriacies might constitute a communicative achievement. What this suggests is that the notion of inappropriacy depends not only on norms and contexts but also on the processing abilities of the client and his/her ability to handle deficiencies. This may present a problem from the observer's point of view in that what he/she requires is in-depth knowledge of the client's communication patterns in order to investigate and make allowances for possible compensatory strategies, which in themselves are not easy to study (Chapter 3). Following Prutting and Kirchner (1987), McTear and Conti-Ramsden (1989) suggest that associating inappropriacy with detrimental effects on interaction enables one to distinguish between inappropriacy which does not result from compensatory strategies and inappropriacy which does. The latter type of inappropriacy has the function of furthering the interaction. Notwithstanding the difficulty in determining what furthers interaction and what does not, the distinction between inappropriacy stemming from the use of communication strategies or some other causes is perhaps a more subtle one. One can think of compensatory strategies such as topic avoidance or even topic shift which may not further the interaction from an observer's point of view but may do so from the client's by indicating willingness to participate at all. Unfortunately for researchers and practitioners, to be able to explore inappropriacy in a clinically useful way, compensatory strategies need to be taken account of, yet how precisely one would do this is not at all clear given that devising a compensatory strategy is an internal operation.

McTear and Conti-Ramsden (1989) explore a further complication with the notion of inappropriacy. A client's communicative partner is also likely to use strategies to compensate for the client's shortcomings. It is not unusual for partners to fake understanding, to paraphrase for the client, to complete his/her utterances, to initiate and respond and to converse on familiar and conceptually simple topics (e.g. Leinonen and Smith, 1989). This may be yet another aspect of inappropriacy/appropriacy which requires further investigation.

This exploration of the notion of appropriacy/inappropriacy ties up with the difficulty of determining the severity of pragmatic disturbance. As was discussed in Chapter 5, pragmatic problems can be approached from different perspectives which in turn may suggest different severity ratings. More specifically, a pragmatic problem might be disturbing in relation to the client's personal and communicative needs or in relation to those interacting with the client. Or, a pragmatic problem might be deemed severe because the very basis of the functioning of the pragmatic component is being affected. A pragmatic problem might also be perceived as disturbing if it is difficult to remediate. There are clearly many different, yet interacting, perspectives from which to observe and assess pragmatic behaviours and of which the clinician needs to be aware.

Before leaving the topic of interpretation of findings and estimation of severity, it may be helpful to consider the concept of fine-grained analysis. It is not sufficient merely to note that certain behaviours are either present or absent, desirable or undesirable. Both clinicians and researchers require more detailed information as to the nature of the behaviours observed and their patterns of occurrence in order to explore pragmatic functioning and form opinions as to the remedial needs of clients. Prutting and Kirchner (1983) propose six parameters for such fine-grained analysis: frequency, latency, duration, density, amplitude/intensity, and sequence.

1. Frequency refers to the number of times a particular behaviour occurs. However, McTear and Conti-Ramsden (1989) question the validity of using frequency of occurrence of behaviours as an index of severity. Behaviours which are not frequent may nevertheless have an adverse effect on communication. They quote the example from Prutting and Kirchner's (1987) case study, where a single behaviour of a client lying down after entering a room has a detrimental effect on the subsequent interaction by demonstrating extreme non-co-operation. While frequency of occurrence of behaviours as a sole indicator of pragmatic disturbance is clearly doubtful, it is likely to tap into some of the oddness of those having

communication problems. It may be that many of the 'inappropriate' behaviours of the 'pragmatically disturbed' do indeed surface in the 'normal' population, but less frequently and, possibly, in different contexts. Further data on this is needed.

2. Latency refers to the time that elapses between a cue and a response, be it appropriate or inappropriate. In relation to the notion of inappropriacy, a behaviour may be judged unacceptable if it does not occur within a 'given' time limit. This tries to capture inappropriately prolonged silences, topics which are not contingently elaborated upon and other such manifestations. The problems with this measure are again clearly visible given the lack of 'norms' and the problem of deciding from whose perspective the latency is being judged. As was discussed in relation to turn-taking in Chapter 3, those feeling anxious when interacting with children or handicapped individuals can easily perceive silences as being long or can eliminate silences by taking the other person's turn.

3. Duration can also run into difficulties because of lack of a point of comparison and yet it quite clearly captures some sense of inappropriacy and severity of disturbance. For instance, how long must eye contact continue before one begins to experience it as inappropriate?

4. Density refers to the frequency of occurrence of behaviours within a given time-span. An utterance or behaviour which may be appropriate on the first occasion of use can become inappropriate if repeated too frequently within a given unit of time.

5. Amplitude/intensity concerns response magnitude. Overloud and exaggerated responses can be experienced as socially inappropriate.

6. Sequence emphasizes the importance of observing chains of interaction rather than focusing on individual behaviours. McTear and Conti-Ramsden (1989) further stress the importance of considering pragmatic assessment as interpersonal. The minimum unit of analysis ought to be that of a dyad, whereas clinical assessment procedures tend to focus on the client. All participants of interactions affect one another in ways that pragmatic

appraisal needs to consider. This point gains further weight if it is acknowledged that it is not always clear which member of a family group should be regarded as 'client'.

Complexity has also been examined as a possible assessment parameter. McTear and Conti-Ramsden (1989) point out the difficulty of grading pragmatic phenomena. Apparently simple pragmatic activity may have involved complex cognitive processes, whereas linguistically complex utterances may be pragmatically unsophisticated. Within linguistic analysis it is well recognized that 'complexity' is likely to reflect theoretical assumptions rather than psychological processes (Chomsky, 1965). Analysis of utterances at one level can produce complexity not evidenced at another (Crystal, Fletcher and Garman, 1976).

FRAMEWORKS FOR ASSESSMENT

Before overviewing specific assessment procedures, some more general characteristics of analytical frameworks need to be discussed. Three main types of assessment approach can be identified: ethnographic approaches; checklists and tests. These are discussed in detail in McTear and Conti-Ramsden (1989) and this discussion need not be restated here. It suffices to note the fundamental features of the ethnographic approach here. The characteristics of checklists and tests will become apparent in the discussion of specific procedures below.

In reaction to linguistic emphasis on language structure, Hymes (1971, 1972b) explored language use in relation to communicative settings, participants and activities. This ethnography of speaking involves identification of groups of speakers constituting a speech community; description of the linguistic resources and styles available for meaning expression and provision of data on setting, participants, purposes, topics, channels of communication and manner of expression. Given the numerous parameters operational in such an undertaking, ethnographic description is essentially qualitative, and impressionistic, rather than quantitative. Ethnography of speaking is also interested in the norms of the speech community and how they may be contravened in different speech events. As such, an ethnographic approach is a descriptive approach to behaviour in naturalistic contexts, dispensing with pre-stated descriptive categories. While such a broad, non-prescriptive, view of communication is valuable in speech therapy, it requires to be supplemented by more focused observational methods (Chapter 4). In this way, attention is directed to specific areas of difficulty in addition to the person's communicative functioning as a whole. Ripich and Spinelli's (1985) approach to assessment and intervention in the classroom illustrates an ethnographic approach to studying children's communication (McTear and Conti-Ramsden, 1989).

OVERVIEW OF PRAGMATIC ASSESSMENT PROTOCOLS

The purpose of this section is to provide an overview of assessment approaches which seek to explore communicative behaviour and the use of language. We aim to inform as to the range of approaches available for different client groups and for different purposes rather than to evaluate the instruments individually. The above discussion on sampling, analysis and interpretation, however, provides some initial guidelines for evaluation. The purpose is to overview approaches suitable for both adult and child populations, though we are less familiar with the field of adult pathology.

Adult learning disability

In the area of adult learning disability (sometimes referred to as mental handicap) many assessments designed for use with child populations can be adapted to provide a valuable picture of communicative development. These approaches will be discussed later.

Wirz (1981) constructed a checklist for the observation of communication skills in learning disabled populations which would be suitable for any age group. It covers a wide range of communicative behaviours which are categorized as follows: expression; listening/comprehension; language usage; articulation; paralinguistic observations and imitation. While some of these categories focus on more traditional areas of speech pathology, more innovative aspects of pragmatic skill are also addressed. It attempts to capture the client's ability to engage in purposeful social activity in different situations and with different partners. It focuses both on verbal and non-verbal (paralinguistic) aspects of communication but, as an early study, did this fairly non-systematically and superficially. The purpose was to provide a useful tool for focusing nurses' and teachers' attention on the communication of their patients and pupils. Some of the issues addressed appear to have become neglected in the more current communication profiles and would be worth further consideration (e.g. exploring the relationship between intonation and intelligibility). The frequency of behaviours is observed and some judgements of appropriacy or inappropriacy of behaviours are also involved.

A more recent method of assessing the communicative abilities of adults with mental handicap (severe to mild) was developed by van der Gaag (1988). The Communication Assessment Profile (CASP) concentrates on verbal behaviour, examining language production, comprehension and use in everyday situations. The functionality of one's communication is explored on the basis of whether the client's skills match the environmental demands. This information is elicited via a questionnaire to be completed by the client's key worker. Being carefully validated in clinical trials involving 350 mentally handicapped adults and 465 speech therapists and care staff, this profile provides a reliable and a relevant measure of communicative ability in this population. It is intended to be used jointly by speech therapists and care staff, thus encouraging integration of skills and views in order to obtain a more realistic understanding of the communicative strengths and weaknesses of the client.

For an up-to-date and comprehensive treatment of issues concerning assessment of communicative behaviours in this client group, the reader is referred to Calculator and Bedrosian (1988).

Adult aphasia

Sarno (1969) challenged the practice of assessing aphasic patients in terms of tests which 'concerned themselves with

identifying "what" the patient said, not "how" he communicated' (p. 1). She developed the Functional Communication Profile (FCP) to explore functional performance
in everyday situations. The FCP consists of 45 behaviours
considered common in everyday urban life: handling money,
speaking on the telephone, greeting. While not being a
sophisticated device, it is based on many solid pragmatic
principles upon which later developed profiles have built.
In their development of the Edinburgh Functional Communication Profile, Skinner, Wirz, Thompson and Davidson
(1984) pointed out that FCP fails to consider communicative
intent and the use of non-verbal communication in different
contexts.

Communicative Abilities in Daily Living (CADL) (Holland,
1980) is a test of functional communication for aphasic
adults. This is a standardized assessment of performance
in role-playing tasks such as telephoning and shopping.
While being a well-motivated research-based assessment
tool, CADL suffers from the limitations imposed by its role-
playing requirements. Only those who function at fairly
high levels can follow complex instructions and engage in
role-playing activities (Skinner *et al.*, 1984). Furthermore,
role-play situations such as visiting the doctor are susceptible to socio-cultural variation. Smith (1985) addresses a
further problem with CADL: are the behaviours assessed
truly those actually needed by aphasic adults? Smith conducted a survey of the communicative needs of dysphasic
adults and found that many of the activities assessed on
CADL were not in fact important for the patients. She
therefore concluded that a standardized test which may con-
tain many irrelevant tasks might not be suitable for assessing functional communication in aphasic adults. She further
suggests that the assessment of the client's communicative
needs ought to be the first stage of pragmatic assessment,
followed by a standardized assessment.

Penn (1988) explores a Profile of Communicative Appropriateness which she developed specifically for use with
adult aphasic patients. It is a profile with a strong discourse analytical dimension (e.g. coherence and cohesion)
in addition to its broadly pragmatic aspects (e.g. fluency,
polite forms, sarcasm/humour). The profile has six main

sections which are divided into eight or so more fine-grained categories. The main categories are those of response to interlocutor (including clarification requests), control of semantic content (namely topical development, including lexical choice), cohesion, fluency, sociolinguistic sensitivity (including direct and indirect speech acts; acknowledgements) and non-verbal communication (including suprasegmental features). The client's behaviours are judged appropriate/inappropriate on a five point scale of appropriacy (inappropriate – mostly inappropriate – some appropriate – mostly appropriate – appropriate) in relation to the 49 individual parameters within the broad categories. It was found in a pilot study that a two-term scale of appropriate–inappropriate produced poor inter-rater reliability and this was rejected in favour of the five-point scale. It is based not only on the notion of appropriacy but also that of frequency.

The Right Hemisphere Language Battery (Bryan, 1989) includes a range of procedures which provide information on impairment of pragmatic and discourse skills of aphasic adults. Contrary to what the name would suggest, this approach addresses communicative rather than linguistic impairment. The procedures are research-based (Bryan, 1988). The battery consists of six sets of tests and a check-list of discourse and pragmatic behaviours for use in exploring a spontaneous sample. Five of the tests examine comprehension (Metaphor Picture Test; Written Metaphor Test; Comprehension of Inferred Meaning; Appreciation of Humour; Lexical Semantic Test) and one production (Production of Emphatic Stress). The Discourse Analysis checklist consists of eleven parameters for assessment (supportive routines, including greetings, thanking etc; humour; questions; assertive routines, including complaining, demanding etc; narrative; variety of topic content, including types of interaction; formality; turn taking; meshing, the timing of the interaction; discourse comprehension; prosody). Behaviours reflecting these parameters are rated on the scale of 0 to 4, 0 reflecting severely limited performance and 4 representing discourse skills within the normal range. The rater is required to make integrated judgements about normality and appropriateness of behaviours, about the potential effect of the client's behaviour on others and about whether or not the limitation was due to aphasia. Although it is not clear how inter-rater reliability could be achieved for such a complex and subjective rating system, it nevertheless draws attention to the importance of investigating discourse and pragmatic skills in this subject population. The sets of tests are also potentially useful in focusing on specific pragmatic skills. What however remains to be shown is, exactly what skills and abilities these tests are attempting to capture. For instance, what does finding that patients have difficulty with non-literal meanings such as metaphor tell us about ability to process information, about underlying knowledge structures and about pragmatic and communicative skill? It is not until we seriously consider such fundamental questions that we can have truly useful assessment protocols. Mean-while, results need to be cautiously interpreted.

Lomas, Pickard, Bester, Elbard, Finlayson and Zoghaib (1989) developed The Communicative Effectiveness Index (CETI) to measure change in the performance of adults with aphasia over time. It aims to provide an instrument to measure functional changes occurring during aphasic patients' recovery process, which have so far eluded measurement. The emphasis is on measuring actual rather than potential performance in daily living. Therefore, the assessment is based on reports from direct observation made of the aphasic individual's communicative functioning by a significant other, a person who spends enough time with the individual to have adequate opportunity to observe. Situations elicited from groups of aphasic patients and their spouses are judged on a visual analogue scale which reflects performance of the individual relative to premorbid ability. At one end of the scale is 'not at all able' and at the other end 'as able as before the stroke'. In order to capture change, performance is rated on a series of different occasions. The raters are encouraged to try to tap into the individual's over-all ability to share meanings with others by whatever means available. In this way verbal communication is not given undue emphasis. The CETI aims to give a realistic account of a person's ability to function in everyday situations and to be flexible and easy to administer. While Lomas *et al.* found the CETI to have accept-able test-retest and inter-rater reliability, further research on its usefulness for researchers and clinicians is currently being undertaken.

For further reading on assessment of this population, Green (1984), Blomert, Koster, van Mier and Kean (1987), Lesser and Milroy (1987) and Rosenbek, LaPointe and Wertz (1989) are recommended.

Childhood communication problems and disorders

When assessing childhood communicative abilities, it is essential to keep in mind that pragmatic performance and potential should take precedence over language skills. This is because specific disorders and difficulties can be com-pensated for and even overcome provided that the child is encouraged to communicate, whereas focusing solely on specific problems may bring about a deterioration in a child's communicative behaviour.

The identification of 'semantic-pragmatic disorder' will not be our primary focus here for reasons which were dis-cussed in Chapter 5. The characteristic behaviours of chil-dren thus classified are overviewed in that chapter and there is no test or assessment battery which reliably incor-porates them into a diagnostic procedure. Awareness of the existence and variety of pragmatic problems should alert teachers and clinicians to the possibility that any child whose speech and language skills are satisfactory but who creates an impression of oddness and inappro-priacy in communicative situations requires further investi-gation by means of some of the methods described in this chapter.

Further reference to Chapter 5 will serve as a reminder that several areas of functioning impinge upon pragma-tic capabilities (e.g. cognitive, neurological, social, linguis-tic). It is the function of the speech-language clinicians to consider areas which they may not be fully trained to as-sess and to refer clients for expert appraisal. The aim here is to discuss only communicatively focused assessment procedures.

Comprehension and semantic functioning

Space does not allow investigation of these complex and important areas. The reader is referred to Chapman (1978), Miller, Chapman, Branston and Reichle (1980), Bishop (1982, 1987), Crystal (1982), Dewart (1989) and Landells (1989). As Bishop (1987) reminds us there are different aspects to comprehension and there are children who appear not to have any problems with comprehension tests such as TROG (Test for the Reception of Grammar, Bishop, 1983) but who have comprehension difficulties in conversation. Such pragmatic comprehension involves integration of many types of information and is likely to be influenced by cognitive, emotional and social factors. This phenomenon requires much further investigation.

Organizational frameworks

Roth and Spekman (1984a) outline areas of pragmatic phenomena which an assessment protocol for children's communicative ability needs to cover. The broad areas are those of communicative intention, presupposition and discourse organization which are further sub-categorized as follows.

1. The assessment of communicative intention (speech acts; Chapter 3) involves analysis of their range and form. Both the variety of intentions expressed and the means by which intention is coded need to be examined.
2. Assessment of presupposition focuses on the child's ability to take the perspective of the communicative partner. This involves assessment of handling of old and new information, of ability to role play and the use of deixis. Sensitivity of a child to the communicative partner can also be examined in relation to social context variables such as communicative demands placed by different partners, situations and channels.
3. By examining the social organization of discourse, one focuses on the child's ability to function in an ongoing stream of interaction. One aims to capture differences between speech used for social purposes and non-social speech such as monologues, individual narratives and

rhymes. Turn-taking, talking time, initiation strategies, adherence to co-operative principles, topical development and conversational repairs are other areas of enquiry.

In addition to considering what to assess, Roth and Spekman (1984b) outline some useful procedures for how to assess the specific areas of pragmatic functioning, both receptive and productive. Familiarity with the details of these important papers will assist in research endeavours and the clinical management of pragmatic problems. Space does not allow an adequate discussion here and thus the reader is advised to refer to the original articles.

Damico (1985) provides a method (Clinical Discourse Analysis) for identifying and describing the communicative problems encountered in children above the age at which he finds language tests to be of value (6 to 8 years). It can also be used in adult assessment. By analysing language samples from 38 language disordered subjects between the ages of 6; 7 and 22; 3, seventeen problem behaviours were identified. These inappropriate behaviours were categorized within Grice's (1975) framework of co-operative maxims (Chapter 1). Failure to provide adequate information to listeners or informational redundancy are examples of violations of the maxim of quantity. The maxim of quality can be compromised by inaccurate messages, while poor topic maintenance and inappropriate response render discourse relationally inadequate (Maxim of Relation). The maxim of manner can become violated by such features as linguistic nonfluency, turn-taking problems and gaze inefficiency. The clustering of problem behaviours under Grice's maxims suggests a basis for identifying common features in apparently unconnected errors. Being concerned with the fundamental co-operative aspect of communication, this framework is even more basic than those based on intentionality and speech acts. Performing a variety of speech acts without adhering to the co-operative principles (and the politeness principle, Chapter 1 and Leech, 1983) is likely to render interactions unsatisfactory. The fact that successful communicators can violate the maxims intentionally for co-operative purposes does present a problem for the categorization of clinical behaviours but not one which cannot be overcome through awareness and common sense.

A further work which contributes to the assessment of communicative function in older children and adults is that of Wiig and Semel (1980). An area of children's pragmatic functioning, which is seldom assessed, that of clarification and repair, is discussed in detail by Brinton and Fujiki (1989) in addition to the more familiar area of turn taking. The latter authors stress the importance of establishing base-lines and availing oneself of information from the client's family by pre-assessment questionnaires such as Gallagher (1983) (see below).

Pre-assessment

Before embarking on any assessment procedure clinicians regularly conduct observational assessments and give consideration to the question of where a client's optimal performance is likely to occur. They also incorporate care-givers at every stage of assessment. One method of systematizing this activity is presented by Gallagher (1983). This Pre-Assessment Questionaire utilizes the care-giver's knowledge of the child's variable behaviour in daily situations to identify the people, materials and situations likely to maximize the child's communicative performance. Such pre-assessment further encourages incorporation of care-givers as members of the assessment team. Since pre-assessment is clearly a socio-culturally specific activity, clinicians may need to design their own questionnaires for specific purposes.

Communicative intention or speech acts

The impetus for much of the attention currently paid to communicative intention in children springs from the shift which occurred in child language studies under the influence of Bates (1974, 1976), Bates, Camaioni and Volterra (1975), Halliday (1975) and Dore (1975). Studies of linguistic development had dominated the field until that time. The focus then moved to the performance of speech acts; the use or attempted use of communicative behaviour to affect the actions or mental states of others (Chapter 3).

Even in the very early stages of development several communicative functions can be identified. Bates (1976) discusses protodeclaratives and protoimperatives as pre-verbal devices for expressing intent. Protodeclaratives serve the function of directing an adult's attention and proto-imperatives function as early requests for action, develop-ing out of children's attempts to do things for themselves. Halliday (1975) identified seven communicative functions in one child's early use of language: instrumental ('I want'); regulatory ('Do as I tell you'); interactional ('Me and You'); personal ('Here I come'); heuristic ('Tell me why'); imagin-ative ('Let's pretend'); informative ('I've got something to tell you'). Instrumental, regulatory, interactional and personal function were observed to develop before heuristic and imaginative, which in turn preceded the informative function. Similarly, Dore (1975) identified a set of primitive speech acts in the one-word utterances of children. These were labelling, repeating, answering, requesting (action), requesting (information), calling, greeting, protesting and practising. Coggins and Carpenter (1981) identified speech acts similar to those of Bates and Dore in pre-verbal (non-verbal) children. Chapman (1981) provides an overview of the above approaches to early childhood intentionality.

Before looking at specific assessment procedures focus-ing on communicative intention, some general observations need to be made. The main problem is that it is not always certain which function or intention should be attributed to an act. For instance is the use of question forms 'heuristic' or 'regulatory'? Is the use of 'Mummy, mummy!' an in-stance of calling or protesting? Much depends upon con-text, knowledge of the child and the pre-disposition of the examiner. The observer's problem in determining speaker-intention arises from:

1. The inherent impossibility of knowing what is in an-other person's mind (McTear, 1985a);
2. The lack of one-to-one correspondence of linguistic form and communicative function;
3. The possibility of one expression carrying more than

one illocutionary force and the possibility of a hierarchy of transparency (e.g. 'hidden meanings and
ulterior motives', Labov and Fanshel, 1977, Chapter 3);
4. The possibility of illocutionary force being negotiated
between participants (Stubbs, 1983, Chapter 3);
5. The constraining effect of social roles and relationships
(e.g. certain acts may not be permitted or welcomed
in specific contexts, Chapter 3);
6. The unpredictability of creative, unusual and original
expressions (e.g. witticisms, jokes);
7. Socio-cultural specificity of interpretation of illocutionary
force;
8. The possibility of a legitimate opting out of performing
speech acts (Bonikowska, 1988, Chapter 3);
9. Unconventional means of expressing illocutionary force
(e.g. requesting by shifting gaze to a desired object,
greeting by waving the foot);
10. Expressions gaining illocutionary force by combination
of verbal and non-verbal means (Chapter 3);
11. The apparent illocutionary force carried by a verbal
expression being contradicted by a non-verbal one.

Despite the difficulties involved in the study of speech
acts, the centrality of intention in the sharing of meaning
cannot be ignored. Provided that the non-absolute quality
of one's attributions of communicative intention is kept in
mind, valuable information about a child's communicative
functioning can be obtained.

Tough (1977a and b) provides a framework for classifying
school-aged children's uses of language. This is a multi-
layered classificatory system where four 'main' functions
(directive, interpretive, projective and relational) are subdivided into two or three more specific functions, which in
turn are divided into even more specific strategies. For
instance, the relational function consists of a self-maintaining
function which in turn consists of subcategories of 'referring to needs', 'projection of self-interest', 'justification'
'criticism' and 'threats'. As a layered approach, the system
enables the observer to capture the relatedness of specific
language functions and also to focus on fairly detailed
communicative acts. The framework can be used both as

a checklist to study children's communicative performance and a framework for setting up teaching situations for facilitating children's use of language. Tough's framework has been used widely by teachers in the UK.

Rather a different approach to children's communicative intent has been developed by Lucas (1980). The Behavioural Inventory of Speech Act Performances (BISAP) is a test which tries to elicit specific acts in the context of art work. In addition to the child, the context for the inventory includes the teacher and another person who makes a judgement about the child's performance, using the categories in the inventory as soon as verbal instructions are given to the child. There are specific tasks which are designed to elicit eight different speech acts. A child has one minute to complete the task after receiving the instructions. An example of a task designed to elicit a request for action would be suggesting to the child that he/she get the teacher to draw a picture. The child's performance is checked against the categories on the BISAP. The structure of the BISAP is based on Searle's (1969) felicity conditions which attempt to specify rules for what makes a specific speech act have the force it does. Such essential elements of speech acts are then specified in the inventory against which the absence or presence of such elements in the child's performance are checked and scored (1 = present; 0 = absent). To illustrate, the following are specified as essential conditions for 'Request for action' (teacher to draw):

1. S's (speaker's/child's) body orientation is toward H (hearer/teacher) in order to ready H for the utterance;
2. Eye contact or name is used to signal H;
3. Appropriate linguistic markers indicating either an interrogative form or imperative form;
4. An utterance which specifies what the H is to do;
5. Appropriate loudness for the H to respond.

Specification of such elements enables one to examine what might contribute towards successful or unsuccessful performance of speech acts. The presence of the elements provides evidence for whether the child is or is not attempting to get the hearer to perform a specific action. Such investigation can be perceived as attempting to specify what a person might need to know in order to perform successful speech acts. This knowledge could be further explored if it was possible to determine whether the child operated with other types of speech act conditions (Preparatory and sincerity rules in Searle, 1969; also Lucas Arwood 1983). As an approach to intentionality, the BISAP is an innovative one in the area of child language pathology. Being a test with a built-in time constraint, the BISAP requires good co-operation and rapid comprehension on the part of the child and thus might be difficult to use with young or poorly functioning children. Also, the scores obtained are of limited value, given that normative data does not currently exist. On the positive side, however, even though the BISAP was designed as a test, the speech act framework can be used for more informal observation of children's communication and as a basis for therapy plans.

Heublein and Bate (1988) describe a method for exploring not only illocutionary force but also perlocutionary effect and the mode of expression (locution). In addition, note is taken of whether or not an illocutionary act is performed (whether behaviours are communicative or non-communicative). Emphasis is placed on describing and analysing the verbal and non-verbal behaviours of all interactants in order to appreciate how children's partners can influence their performance. Having identified and categorized the behaviours, frequencies and patterns of behaviour are determined. This is in order to establish whether the balance of contributions from each partner is heavily weighted in one direction and whether a range of types of acts is employed. Both partners are likely to influence the range of intentions expressed by the other. For instance, a minimally communicative partner may prompt the other to ask many questions, while the excessive questioning may in turn encourage minimal contribution. The procedure also requires some judgements to be made about the successfulness of the attempted communicative acts. Exploration of the behaviour patterns with care-givers is also encouraged. The procedure enables the clinician to devise comprehensive treatment plans and to monitor progress which compensates for the time-consuming nature of such a thorough investigation. Weiss' (1981) discussion of the INREAL system (Interactive Learning) also focuses on a comprehensive analytical framework for dyadic interaction.

The Interactive Record (Smith, 1987) provides a means of exploring dyadic, or even group, interaction. By enabling one to record and analyse the communicative contributions of all interactants, it reveals the possible effects of people upon one another, thus acknowledging the shared responsibility for communication. Data is transcribed directly onto a record sheet outlining the analytical categories. This provides a method of retrieving information at a glance and a means of cross-checking different analyses and interpretations of what has occurred. The present analytical framework focuses on intention and perlocution in addition to noting manner of expression and contextual information. A revised version is currently being developed.

Wetherby and Prizant (1989) provide useful guidelines for the assessment of communicative intent in children. While much of their discussion is fairly general, addressing issues in sampling and interpretation, it highlights the need for both 'horizontal and vertical dimensions' in assessment of intentional communication. The horizontal dimension involves assessment of 'the variety and range of functions and intents expressed' and the vertical dimension involves assessment of 'the level of intentionality and the sophistication of means that are relative to specific communicative functions' (p. 83). Specific categories, based on normal developmental literature, for assessing both of these dimensions are provided. For examining the range of communicative functions categories similar to those of Halliday (1975) and Dore (1975) are included. In relation to the vertical dimension one is looking for evidence for the child using signals to have a preplanned or intentional effect on the behaviour of others, thus enabling one to examine metapragmatic awareness. The framework for exploring this vertical dimension includes categories such as 'Awareness of a goal', 'Simple plan designed to achieve a goal' and 'Alternative plans designed to achieve a goal'. Wetherby and Prizant discuss briefly some procedures which can be used to test hypotheses about intentionality.

The extent to which these procedures will provide information about underlying intention remains to be demonstrated.

The Affective Communication Assessment (Coupe, Barton, Barber, Collins, Levy and Murphy, 1985) is an approach to investigating the intentionality of non-verbal behaviours in pre-verbal severely learning disabled children. A checklist of bodily activities is provided (e.g. Head/ rotating; Mouth/tongue activity; Hands/finger activity), in relation to which communicative intent is interpreted. The procedure involves the observer selecting stimuli, to which the child is already known to respond. The non-verbal responses are then assigned an interpretation which is assumed to reflect affective communication (i.e. the child is interpreted as trying to communicate). For example, using this procedure a child has been observed to respond consistently to a familiar song and certain adult activities by laughing, vocalizing, smiling and by increased hand and finger activity. These are interpreted as expressing liking of the activities. It is pointed out that most functions which appear to be expressed are those of 'I want/I don't want' or 'I like/I don't like'. By relating adult stimuli to child behaviour and subsequent interpretation, the assessment takes some account of the interpersonal nature of communication. It also enables one to find a starting point for working with individuals so severely handicapped that they might otherwise be deemed totally non-communicating.

WIDE-RANGING OBSERVATIONAL CHECKLISTS

The checklist approach to pragmatic assessment is considered in this section. Many of these lists include intention and speech acts but range more widely over the features of pragmatic ability in an attempt to alert teachers, therapists and researchers to strengths and shortcomings which might otherwise be ignored. When gaps in performance become evident in this way, it cannot be assumed that similar gaps in ability exist; further investigation is called for. Checklists are not devices for investigating causes and motivations for behaviours but rather for organizing one's observations. Therefore, sub-categories of behaviours tend to be related at a superficial level (e.g. using language for a purpose) rather than sharing some more fundamental similarity (e.g. involving the handling of extended discourse or the politeness principle). Checklists vary in design and coverage depending on the purpose and theoretical orientation of their authors and therefore it is helpful to be aware of the range that is available.

On the basis of Johnston's (1980) Communication Abilities Test, Johnston, Weinrich and Johnson (1984) developed a checklist for exploring the level of adequacy of children's pragmatic functioning. The Pragmatic Observations List covers various communicative behaviours which are judged adequate or inadequate. In addition to the more usually included speech act categories (e.g. Can the child use language to ask for help, label objects, pretend and greet people?), the checklist also includes exploration of language functions such as using language for making choices, for telling stories, for expressing needs and feelings and for 'talking about talking' (metalinguistics). The checklist also focuses on whether a child can produce different sentence types (e.g. negatives, interrogatives etc.), or produces contextually relevant, adequately informative, polite and truthful language (cf. Grice, 1975). Further questions involve establishment of eye contact, handling of exchange structure, turn taking and topical development. Described as such, this procedure appears to cover a wide range of conversational ability and skill but because it is simply a checklist, guidance for interpreting the significance of the observations is not provided.

Another assessment procedure designed to be used with pre-verbal severely learning disabled populations is Kiernan and Reid's (1987) Pre-Verbal Communication Schedule. Six aspects of communicative functioning are examined: attention seeking; need satisfaction; simple negation; positive interaction: negative interaction; shared attention. The schedule is intended not only for child populations but for those who are pre-verbal or with very limited verbal ability. While it is primarily a checklist of behaviours, the frequency of which is noted, it also consists of some test items for examining motor imitation and understanding of non-vocal communication. It tries to differentiate between behaviours which are intentionally communicative and those which are not. Sections on pre-communicative behaviours, informal communicative behaviours and formal communication skills address this distinction. While adequate inter-rater reliability was found, the difficulty of assigning or not assigning intentionality to non-verbal behaviours must be appreciated. A further distinction is made between communication by non-verbal means and by symbolic systems such as verbal or signed language. The usefulness of pooling information from different sources such as parents, care-workers or nurses is emphasized. Consisting of 195 items, the schedule can take more than two hours to complete. It however enables one to investigate the beginnings of communicative functioning and is designed to assist in extending the limited use made of small communicative repertoires.

Prutting and Kirchner's (1983) Pragmatic Protocol (see also Prutting and Kirchner, 1987; Kirchner and Prutting, 1989) is a widely used, comprehensive checklist of pragmatic skills. The over-all organization of the checklist is based on speech act theory (though it is not clear precisely how) reflecting its centrality in the shift from grammatical theory to theory of language use. The protocol is divided into three main sections. 'Utterance act' covers the verbal, paralinguistic and non-verbal means of expressing intention. 'Propositional act' includes categories such as lexical selection and use, word order, given/new information and stylistic variation. The section on 'illocutionary and perlocutionary acts' covers a wide range of behaviours such as speech acts, topic and turntaking. The way in which the behaviours are grouped within a speech act framework is not clear, nor does it enable one to clarify the nature of a client's underlying difficulties. The behaviours are judged as appropriate or inappropriate in relation to whether or not they are communicatively penalizing to the client. Despite its organizational shortcomings, the protocol provides a method of identifying many of a client's communicative strengths and weaknesses and how these alter over time. The protocol provides a broad analysis which can be supplemented by finer-grain examinations on the lines suggested by Prutting and Kirchner (1983) (see above).

McTear (1985a) provides a checklist of discourse skills. This is a means of profiling conversational ability under the categories of turn taking, initiation, response, cohesion and repairs. McTear considers this as a preliminary checklist since the construction of a developmental profile would be premature. While the overall framework is based on discourse analytical categories, limited accounts of speech act types (i.e. attention-getters; attention-directors) and mode of expression (attention-getting: verbal or non-verbal) are included. Each of the categories is analysed in relation to the frequency of occurrence of behaviours. In relation to responses, judgements of appropriacy are made.

The Pragmatics Profile of Early Communication Skills by Dewart and Summers (1988) is an interview schedule attempting to describe the child's typical communicative behaviours in a variety of settings. Information in the areas of communicative functions, response to communication, manner of participation and the effect of different settings on communicative functioning is obtained from care-givers in a semi-structured interview. Based on broad functional categories, the profile is suitable for both normal and language impaired children, being specifically valuable for exploring the functioning of those with little or no language. The profile alerts both clinicians and care-givers to the child's attempted communications, and to the influence of others upon how the child interacts. It can also reveal to clinicians how the child is perceived by different individuals and what range of experiences and communicative opportunities is available for the child. It is also considered useful in assessing the pragmatic skills of children from different cultural backgrounds who may be experiencing difficulty with linguistic communication.

The Bristol Language Development Scales (Gutfreund, 1989) enable language samples to be analysed in terms of syntax, semantics and pragmatics in order to assess levels of development and identify gaps and deficiencies in the use of expressive language. The scales are intended for use with children aged 15 months to 5 years. Being based on a large-scale study of normal development of expressive language, detailed developmental norms are provided. A valuable 'syntax-free' scale is also included for use with non-English speakers, deaf children and those with learning difficulties.

Because of the inherent variability of communicative be-haviours, pragmatic assessment checklists can only reveal what fortuitously occurs. For this reason, tests and probes are used to explore specific areas of functioning. By formu-lating and testing hypotheses, information about poss-ible underlying causes for inadequate functioning can be gathered. Large-scale standardization of pragmatic tests might be possible for well-defined areas of functioning, which reflect basic pragmatic knowledge (Chapter 5) rather than context-dependent behaviours. The problem of the differences in one's performance in test and non-test situa-tions is exaggerated in pragmatic tests but can be counter-acted by focusing on very specific aspects of functioning. In the clinical situation, observational checklist and test/ probe approaches supplement one another.

Blank and Marquis (1987) provide a procedure, which lies in between a checklist and a test, for eliciting informa-tion about discourse and linguistic processes. 20 demands such as 'Find one just like this', 'Tell me what you do with a net' and 'How can we tell if the gelatine is ready?' are presented to the child. The procedure is a checklist in that pre- and post-treatment responses are judged as satisfac-tory or unsatisfactory, and it has features of a test in that a pre-determined set of behaviours is investigated in a one-to-one elicitation setting. The procedure is not stan-dardized. The aim is to facilitate the preparation of indi-vidualized educational plans (IEP) in relation to explicit teaching methods. The checklist is reproducible and a pre-determined format for the IEP is provided. The actual elici-tation of behaviours takes 15–20 minutes.

The Bus Story, The Test of Continuous Speech (Renfrew, 1969) provides a means of investigating some aspects of children's ability to reconstruct narrative discourse. It was designed to be used in conjunction with other linguistic assessments. Bishop and Edmondson (1987) found scores on the bus story test to be the best predictors of whether or not a child's 'language disorder' would resolve by age 5;6. An age range of 3;0–8;0 (265 British children) was covered in the standardization. A story is read to a child who follows a picture version throughout. The child is then asked to retell the story as accurately as possible using the picture version as a prompt. The retelling is then scored for information and average number of words in the five longest sentences (A5LS). The two scores are then compared and inferences suggested. For instance, if the Information Score is more than three and a half times the A5LS, specific difficulties in sentence construction should be investigated. If the A5LS is more than twice the Information Score, specific word finding difficulty might be suspected.

It is realized that narrative skill and the production of continuous speech cannot be fully assessed by means of a memorized and visually prompted retelling. However, these abilities may be central to confident personal use of language; both for thinking and for communication (Nelson, 1989). As yet there are no widely used assessments of these skills. Thus there is a need to develop awareness of their importance and to devise methods of assessing them (see discussion by Westby, Van Dongen and Maggart, 1989). It will also be necessary to investigate the question of whether lack of overt narrative skill represents a limitation in connected thinking or in the transformation of thoughts into connected discourse.

The Test of Pragmatic Skill by Shulman (1985) is an attempt to provide a standardized assessment of pragmatic behaviour suitable for three- to eight-year-olds. The test has been standardized using a sample of 650 children of 3;0–8;11. Shulman is aware that it represents only an initial step in this direction and that variability of behaviour in variable contexts constitutes a major obstacle to accurately assessing an individual's capabilities. What such a test can do however is to demonstrate what an individual is able to perform satisfactorily in a specific situation. As with any test, what cannot be assumed is that children who perform poorly in the test are not capable of doing better in other circumstances. Shulman's test examines ten conversational intentions: requesting information, requesting action, rejection/denial, naming, labelling, answering/responding, informing, reasoning, summoning/calling, greeting and closing conversation. The child's performance as both speaker and listener is systematically observed during two verbal and 'less-verbal' interactive events (i.e. telephone interaction; puppet play; building and design copying). Scores of nought to five are assigned to the child's performance ranging from 0 for no response to contextually appropriate response with extensive elaboration (more than three words) which scores 5. It is not made clear how one is intended to estimate the appropriateness of such elaboration. This is problematic in that a well-functioning child might provide an economical, elliptical response, whereas one whose conversational style could be described as 'pompous' would be likely to provide excessive elaboration.

McTear and Conti-Ramsden (1989) and King (1989) discuss the strengths and weaknesses of the Test of Pragmatic Skills on the following lines. It is helpful to have tests which are easy and quick to administer, which probe a range of communicative intentions and which do not depend too heavily upon verbal ability. These begin to provide valuable norms for pragmatic development. They can be used in conjunction with more naturalistic assessments to confirm or challenge the impressions held by clinicians and other adults about a child's abilities and to investigate particular areas of development. Care must be taken in using tests, such as the Shulman, however, to recognize intentions of the child which are not predicted by the test; to remember that individual assessments of appropriateness vary; to allow for cultural effects and to acknowledge that the clinician's role vis-à-vis the child may forbid certain assertive acts on the part of the child which have been expected (predicted) in the test. Certainly one should maintain an awareness that although certain child-like activities may be described as 'play' the fact that the clinician is in control of the activity, as in the Shulman test, is likely to affect the outcome by limiting both the range of the activity and the child's personal commitment to it, thus restricting the range of intentions that will be expressed.

The Pragmatics Screening Test (Prinz and Weiner, 1987) is designed to be used in conjunction with a Pragmatics Teacher Ratings Scale (not to rate the teacher but to obtain guidance as to how the child should be approached and the results interpreted). The age range of 3;6–8;6 is catered for. A Pre-Test, which is part of the Screening Test, attempts to prepare the child and to provide additional indications as to the child's suitability for the procedure. Scoring and analysis are undertaken not by the tester but by the publishers, on the basis of coded records. This is a disadvantage in that one does not know how to evaluate the analysis. Detailed description of this test can be found in McTear and Conti-Ramsden (1989).

Simon's (1986) Evaluating Communicative Competence: A Functional Pragmatic Procedure seeks to keep syntactic training in its proper perspective by including a wide variety of communicative tasks in a prompted interview-type investigation. This procedure, which is based on wide-ranging observation and reading and on a study of the performance of 25 'good communicators', falls in-between a test and a checklist approach, by relying on probes but not being standardized. It is suitable for school-aged children. Reproducible result tables are provided. This system should be considered together with Simon (1980) and might well provide additional treatment indications for clinicians and teachers working in language units and special schools.

SUMMARY

As this overview shows, assessment of clients' communicative functioning, their pragmatic skills, has become a common enterprise in the clinical context. Emphasis has shifted from considering language skills to looking at the ability to function in everyday situations. Many of the approaches focus on the presence or absence of certain communicative behaviours and on their perceived appropriacy or inappropriacy. Both observational protocols and more structured elicitation techniques are used. Pragmatic tests for more focused exploration of skills are also being developed.

Much of current assessment concentrates on the description of communicative manifestations with the apparent aim of describing some communicative handicap. Given the professional focus of speech-language clinicians, other possible causes of unsatisfactory communication may be overlooked. It is therefore essential to consider the question of whether impaired pragmatics should be regarded purely as an indication of personal short-comings ('the remediable deficit view') or as a disturbance of social functioning and thus a possible indicator that all is not well in the client's life. The current literature on speech pathology tends to focus on deficits, disorders and problems, often to the exclusion of the social circumstances in which they occur. It is dangerously easy to assume that the more extreme clients' behaviour appears, the more likely they are to have an inherent disorder.

The cases of Kimberley Carlile (Blom-Cooper, 1987) and Jasmine Beckford (Blom-Cooper, 1985), both of whom were killed at home and both of whom were referred to speech therapy, highlight the need for a broad view of communication problems and their causes. Jasmine Beckford was reported to be 'behind with her speech' but there was 'no concern' (pp. cv and cxiii). Kimberley Carlile was referred when her mother reported to her family doctor that she was 'not speaking properly'. Social workers noted her 'behavioural problems' including withdrawal, screaming, temper tantrums and wetting. The speech therapy referral was never taken up by her family. Interestingly, in her short-term foster home, Kimberley had been described as a chatterbox, with quite a remarkable vocabulary for her age, as happy, extraverted and conscientious in everything she did. Kimberley died after prolonged torture and starvation by her parents. The report on these events makes salutary reading, giving rise to the question: had Kimberley been presented for speech therapy assessment, would the area review committee have been alerted at that point to the distress the child was experiencing or would the speech therapy department have appeared in the report together with several others as being implicated in her death?

Chapter 7

Issues in treatment

Now that clinicians are learning to recognize problems which involve semantic and pragmatic knowledge and skills, the question of what to do about such problems is uppermost. One hears appeals from all sides for descriptions of pragmatics-based therapy methodology which will transcend the language-programme approach and yet incorporate the known value of established practices. This chapter can be seen as a preliminary response to such appeals. Quite commonly it is asserted that therapy which is based upon a language programme or curriculum or upon the teaching of specific tasks is 'structured', whereas pragmatics-based therapy is 'unstructured'. This is misleading. It is true that one of the most noticeable differences between the two approaches is the degree of autonomy granted to the client. However, the clinician who relinquishes tight control of therapy sessions in order to facilitate the client's active participation does not abandon structure; it is simply that the structure is a looser, negotiable one.

A therapy session might be structured to include the following six steps

1. Planning and preparation;
2. Greeting and conversation and/or play;
3. Oral gymnastics;
4. Rhymes or poetry, possibly with amplified input;
5. Conversation, story or play;
6. Leave-taking and therapeutic summing-up plus suggestions for home activity.

The first of these steps involves the evaluation of assessments and reports; selecting equipment; preparing 'homework'; devising events and problems for the client to wrestle with later (e.g. sabotaging scissors with sticky tape so that the child is motivated to complain; Lucas, 1980); hiding toys; and making arrangements for visits. This structuring stage is highly demanding professionally and, as with 'free' classroom teaching, is crucial to success. If not tailored accurately to the individual client's needs, such preparation will undermine communication rather than facilitate it. Steps two and five are partially under the control of the client and are designed to provide the context for what needs to be learned at any particular stage. Corrections and suggestions can be offered in pragmatics-based therapy, contrary to popular belief, but they should not disrupt the communicative event unduly. Such corrections would also be of short duration and of obvious relevance to the client's concerns. For instance, one might say 'That would be a lot easier to understand if you said it like this . . .', thus demonstrating genuine interest and providing motivation for change. Step three represents the type of brief speech or language drill which many clients require. Step four represents planned input. Step six involves thinking on one's feet about the appropriate summarizing of what has been achieved in the session, what should be attempted before the next session, what should be particularly remembered etc. This stage may also be perceived as an opportunity for giving attention to clients' escorts or relatives who frequently make use of it as counselling time.

Throughout programmes of this nature, the clinician has clear-cut, professional objectives. It may be necessary to express aims in behavioural terms: 'The client shall ask questions. The client shall complain. The client shall request, exclaim, draw attention to'. A more mentalistic aim is likely to be that the client shall enjoy a relationship which provides motivation for learning the rules of language and principles of interaction.

It is somewhat ironic that, having been asked for twenty years how on earth clinicians managed to work without knowledge of linguistics, older professionals are now becoming aware that those fundamental facilitative methods which they were taught as students and which served well clinically are once again in demand. Indeed, it was one of the early writers in speech pathology, Mildred Freburg Berry (1969; also Berry and Eisenson, 1956), who devised in 1980 a Global-Ontogenic teaching programme which states clearly many of the principles we would wish to include in a pragmatically aware treatment manual. We recommend it and also Craig (1983) as starting points for the understanding of pragmatics in therapy.

We shall explore in this chapter how the knowledge of pragmatics can assist the mobilization, acquisition and recovery of skills and how this knowledge helps clinicians to ensure that clients are able to use their skills in real life contexts. The concept of 'pragmatism' is also useful in a more general sense for the speech pathologist. 'Clinical pragmatism' would involve choosing, regardless of tradition or previous belief, strategies which appear to work. Just how disturbing such a policy can be to traditionalists is paralleled by the horror with which many thinkers reacted to philosophical theories of pragmatism which suggested that words could be made to mean whatever human beings needed them to mean, since they had no independent validity of their own (Aune, 1970). To be accused of 'pragmatism' was at one time a serious matter. The term could be used to describe one who behaved in a totally atheoretical manner, who flouted or disregarded high principles, moral systems or established custom in favour of practical gains. Such behaviour was by no means always heroic or altruistic. 'Mere pragmatism' is an expression reserved for exploits or dubious ventures which seem likely to result in gains for the perpetrator, or in short-term success at the expense of long-term integrity. Arguments still rage fiercely as to whether or not moral principles are of any value in circumstances where they can never be put to use due to impracticality. For instance, in a democracy, should a political party cling to idealistic policies which deter people from voting for them? Should clinicians persist with tightly structured therapy, when an interactive approach may be more effective? The sense in which pragmatism is at its most constructive is that which implies neither long- nor short-term gains with neither personal nor altruistic goals, but simply the application of knowledge and common sense to achieve realistic ends, without undue reference to preestablished systems of thought. Experimentation with combinations of approaches might provide insight as to the most effective methods of treatment.

How then are clinicians to become or remain pragmatic in their approach to disordered communication and how are they to employ the insights gained through the study of communicative pragmatics? In an attempt to begin to frame responses to these major questions, some general issues will now be examined.

EFFECTIVENESS AND LIMITATIONS OF ESTABLISHED METHODS OF TREATMENT

For many types of communication problem, treatment effectiveness has not been researched. This makes comparison of methods difficult. There are several reasons for lack of research including shortage of clinical time, lack of funding and traditions of service which preclude the prioritization of research and deter clinicians from seeing themselves as researchers. Other professionals who might be in a stronger position to fill this gap have so far shown little interest in doing so. We see no reason why linguists, psychologists and others would not find it rewarding to address practical issues such as this. Where research has been carried out it is fraught with misunderstandings, misconceptions and terminological difficulties (Russell and Gibson, 1985, Leonard, 1987, Eastwood, 1988). Even the comparatively well researched area of 'language disorder' has run into difficulties (Friel-Patti and Conti-Ramsden, 1984, Leonard, 1987) (Chapter 5).

Leaving such considerations temporarily aside however, it is appropriate to remind readers that in a wide-ranging review of research into the facilitation of language development Leonard (1981) revealed that, on the whole, skills and language forms which had been taught in a rigid and clinic-bound manner did not generalize well to other contexts and that the subjects of such teaching did not experiment with the use of what had been taught. This influential review prompted many clinicians and researchers to pursue the question of how better generalization could be achieved and it was suggested by many, including Smith (1988,

1989), that greater understanding and application of pragmatics might provide answers.

It soon became clear that two major factors were affecting both clinical practice and research into communication problems; one was the excessive focus on 'language' which had occurred during the period of rapid development of linguistic science and its introduction to therapeutic and educational thinking (Crystal, 1972, Quirk, 1972, Smith, 1989). Helpful as the knowledge of language can be, it is not the whole story where human communication is concerned. The other major influence was behaviourism which directed clinicians' attention to observable behaviour, its change and management, with little reference to thoughts, feelings or internal states (see Operant Learning Theory, below). Behaviourism, appropriately applied, has helped many people to take their place in society and to overcome serious difficulties, but as a view of human nature and potential, it has just the sort of limitations to bring about blinkered research and therapy. For example, research which merely examines the improvement or deterioration in a treated, or untreated, patient's tendency to utter certain linguistic forms correctly can be valuable, but only if all concerned are aware that it reveals only a small part of a picture that is larger and more complex. Teaching or therapy can also become limited as a result of narrow linguistic or behaviourist thinking. For instance, it is sometimes assumed that what is needed is training in the production of specific language forms or behaviours rather than the experience of challenging interactions and assistance in equipping oneself with appropriate repertoire and understanding so as to be able to participate. The assumptions made about what needs to be learned will affect judgements about results.

Effectiveness of therapy, then, is a matter which can be judged differently depending on one's philosophy and expectations. For present purposes, we are taking the view that therapy is effective if the client experiences enhanced self-esteem and confidence in communicative situations and if people interacting with the client perceive the interactions as more successful than in the period prior to therapy. These criteria would not be met for all clients in speech pathology at present even if their percentage of correct utterances increased and it is for such clients that insights from pragmatics may be helpful. It is our contention that clients too often remain in the clinical system for long periods making slow progress, when they could be progressing more rapidly toward more personally relevant goals. The fact that some progress can be demonstrated is used to justify the aims and methods selected, whereas, because of insufficient research, it is not known whether faster improvement would be possible. It might be difficult to justify teaching a specific linguistic structure for six months, if conclusive proof that it could be taught in six weeks to similar clients became widely publicized.

ACCOUNTABILITY

Clinicians have always felt accountable to clients and are currently, in the UK, encountering increasing pressures to be accountable to administrative bodies. Clinicians in the USA have always had to deal with these pressures (Chapter 9). For the moment it may be acceptable to justify provision of therapy on the basis of behavioural studies and language-confined assessments (e.g. Reynell; LARSP; Northwestern Syntax; phonological profiles and articulation tests). However, what if the pressure for accountability were to gather further weight and were at the same time to become consumer-led? This would necessitate a move to more personally relevant and socially advantageous treatment. The results of treatment would then have to be differently assessed.

ATTITUDES TO DISABILITY

In moving toward pragmatically based treatment, speech and language clinicians find themselves in line with a movement toward the emancipation of people who have physical or mental illnesses or disabilities. This movement is part of a larger trend which dates from at least the mid-eighteenth century and has empowered successive groups of previously subjugated people. Gradually as the demand for rights and liberty has spread, colonial people, the enslaved, 'the poor', women, the racially oppressed, the physically or mentally different and the physically or mentally ill have begun to be seen as deserving human rights. At times, opposition to emancipation has been violent and determined, while assistance and encouragement have been offered from other quarters. Within each previously oppressed group there is usually dissent, some members wishing to progress and some wishing to retain the advantages of a known and understood regime. The interaction of internal and external forces has always been complex and the effects unpredictable and difficult to evaluate. As a result of experience some of the mechanisms of oppression and liberation are now beginning to be understood; others await clarification. It is known, for instance, that dominant groups impose their own standards when judging oppressed groups e.g. men value strength and tend to judge women as inferior because they are physically less strong. It is known that the oppressed people themselves tend to perpetuate the oppression. It is known that consciousness-raising tends to be effective and that legislation and mutual support can be helpful ('You can't treat me like that. My brother says I should report you.').

The attitudes and beliefs which clinicians or researchers hold with regard to disability in general are likely to be reflected in their work. This is the case even, or perhaps especially, when the attitudes and beliefs are not consciously recognized. What people who are different from the majority, or who are not able to perform as expected complain about in the, currently, able-bodied is an assumption of superiority and a tendency to advise and to make decisions from that assumed position without reference to their experience and wishes. Respect is a commodity which people who are 'different' find difficult to come by, despite widespread eagerness by others to help and to interfere with their lives. A striking example is that of the deaf who for many years were not consulted in the 'oralism' vs. 'signing' controversy despite the fact that implementation of one policy or the other in schools profoundly influenced deaf peoples' lives. After moving gradually from the position of helpless child to respected adult one is capable of understanding how much difference respect can make to the way one feels about life and oneself, and also to the way one approaches other people and the tasks and problems of living. What is problematic is that respect customarily has to be earned, in the sense that one demonstrates one's capability and is then treated differently. Casting our minds back however, many of us are aware that we felt capable before we had proved ourselves and were discouraged or annoyed by the attitudes of those who treated us as incapable or of no account. Furthermore, we rose to the occasion when someone treated us as able to decide for ourselves or asked our opinion and listened to the reply. When given responsibility most of us experience a mixture of fear and joy but cope better than our detractors had expected. The desire for autonomy is strong in human beings and it is with pride and satisfaction that most people embrace it when the opportunity arises.

So far so good. Respect can be seen as a beneficial attitude which many more people ought to experience. Treating others respectfully is not without its problems. However, giving more responsibility to ill or disabled people can be risky. Having genuine weaknesses, areas of ignorance, limited capacity, and competing motivations, like everybody else, they tend to make mistakes. Responsibility can be heavy for them; their opinion may be of limited value and their decisions unwise; they may be simply unable to rise to an occasion or to perform as they would wish particularly in the early stages of coping with a disability. These are the facts which give rise to the custom of witholding respect until proofs of ability are seen. Clearly some active rethinking is required if witholding respect fails to bring out the best in large numbers of human beings. Certainly it is resented and resisted and it may, in fact, serve to suppress abilities which lie dormant and unrecognized until given the opportunity to develop. Where these issues are concerned, negotiation and experimentation may be fraught with risk but may provide a way forward. The disability-rights movement offers help, information and support for this very reason.

Guidelines and principles for interacting with previously disregarded people, such as those with severe learning disabilities will be found in the next section which deals with inter-age-group attitudes because treatment of the young is fundamental to the treatment of any other person who can be seen as 'like a child' and therefore unworthy of respect. A relevant problem here is the widespread insensitivity reported in connection with 'normalization' projects. While excellent in principle such projects have at times resulted in the sudden and fundamentally disrespectful removal of child-like features from the lives of mentally handicapped people. The consequent distress, deprivation and loss of developmental opportunity, in the form of play, is not always acknowledged.

ATTITUDES TO THE YOUNG AND THE OLD

It is now recognized that children and old people are, in many cultures, the recipients of oppressive attitudes on the part of more powerful age groups. Earning power, sexual attractiveness, physical independence and involvement in productive society are usually assumed to confer status. It follows, therefore, that those outside the normal, working population are easily seen as naturally inferior and find themselves ignored, bullied and treated with a lack of consideration that would lead higher status persons to register the strongest possible complaint. Elderly people of independent means escape this treatment to some extent but are not immune, since it is the general view of an age-group's capabilities which holds sway. Both in Britain and the US people beyond retirement age are beginning now to form associations (e.g. 'Grey Panthers'; 'Grey Power') to resist status erosion and to make their wishes and views known. However, the combination of aged appearance and physical frailty is still likely to involve an uphill struggle for dignity and respect.

Very young people are in an even worse position than the old. Almost everyone agrees that it is right and proper for them to be controlled, punished and deprived of choice. Many people regard their wishes as insignificant and underestimate their abilities (Miller, 1981). Others treat them with rudeness, harshness or minor cruelty as a matter of course, feeling little or no remorse because after all they are only children and everyone knows that if one is not hard on 'kids' they get out of line. Imagine applying this thinking to women in the present climate and then recall that it is only some thirty years ago that it was extremely common to do so. What has been described so far is not even major cruelty, neglect or abuse; yet it is now known that these extremes are common and that western societies mistreat their children on a scale unappreciated until recently. When young people are treated well they are frequently seen as 'spoilt' and over-indulged which can often be the case. Their problem is that few of us are clear about the rights that we wish to accord to the young. However, the United Nations Organization has recently adopted a new charter for children which should clarify matters considerably. The United Nations Convention on the Rights of the Child (1989) includes the following provisions: the State must ensure that children receive the highest standard of health care and special assistance if disabled; the State must protect children from all forms of abuse and from any form of discrimination. Furthermore, children have a right to leisure, play, cultural and artistic activities and have the right to make their feelings and views known and to have their opinions taken into account. All rights apply to all children without exception. The convention forms part of international law and has, to date, been notified by 98 countries. It is worth noting that in Britain in 1989 the National Society for the Prevention of Cruelty to Children found it necessary to write the following (in a campaign poster): 'many peoples' (and organizations') attitudes to children need to change. This applies to professionals as well as parents. Often with the best intentions, children are treated without regard for their feelings and opinions rather than as people in their own right'.

As with other attitudes, clinicians do well to examine theirs toward younger and older people, since clinical decisions and style will reflect them. Regardless of their relatively dependent status, the old and the young are entitled to the consideration due to all human beings. This consideration involves thinking about them, attending to their messages, regarding their comfort and safety as no less important than our own and recognizing that, when their desires and ours conflict, automatic supremacy is not one of our rights.

This question of rights is an important one and forms the basis of much of the work currently done in assertiveness training. Such training can also be offered to children in parallel with social skills training. It is viewed somewhat differently in different countries, a fact which gives rise to considerable discussion and argument at the present time (Franklin, 1986). In those rare situations where the rights of all are clearly stated there is less likelihood that fundamentally decent treatment will be regarded as a privilege to be removed or denied at the whim of someone more powerful, though of course it does happen. For instance the elderly stroke patient who asked her speech therapist to remind her sons that she was a 'human person' was perhaps lucky to find one who could (a) understand what she had to say and (b) robustly take her part.

Conflicts of rights and interests happen all the time, yet there is no valid reason why the wishes of the strongest group should always prevail, except that they can enforce them. Preferring not to use power in this way remains an option until the weak are able to band together and acquire power of their own. Sharing power with the old and the young is an option which the present authors have chosen in the same way that many educators and medical experts have chosen to share power with their consumers. This does not mean that all decisions have to be handed over or that one's own interests must be ignored. What it does mean is that we agree to pool our resources to discover what makes sense. It means that we shall give information rather than compel or manipulate others to behave in certain ways and that when it seems necessary to use compulsion, as it must in the case of children at times, we recognize their right to express anger without being punished or reprimanded. Also we should try to treat people courteously, not using their age, or (apparent) lack of ability as an excuse not to do so. We expect them equally to listen to us and to treat us in reasonable ways, though it is possible that some time may elapse before they are able to do this. When either party behaves unreasonably the other has a right to complain. The point at issue is the use of power to control and thus weaken others.

There are certain behaviours which can signify disrespect and might be experienced as humiliating by disadvantaged groups. These behaviours include: witholding resources to which they feel they have a legitimate claim; witholding information or giving misleading or incomprehensible information; witholding responsibility or giving responsibility for which they are not prepared; demanding unrealistic achievement or conversely, making it clear that low expectations are held; stereotyping; patronizing behaviour; intrusiveness and the denial of privacy; coercion; punishment and 'fobbing off'. Furthermore, there can be an offensive attitude which justifies all or any of the above insulting behaviours as for the ultimate good of the recipients (Miller, 1983).

Life certainly proceeds smoothly for the dominant groups when they hold complete control. It can even be argued that members of the less powerful groups do benefit in some ways from the security and freedom from responsibility which this entails. Since the issues are difficult ones to deal with and to resolve professionally we include some references which might prove helpful (Rogers, 1969, Hemmings, 1972, Pringle, 1975, Stallibrass, 1977, Holt, 1982, 1984, Strike, 1982, Pugh and De'Ath, 1984, Elliot, 1985a,b, Gribble, 1985, Rose and Black, 1985, Burgess, 1986, Franklin, 1986, Lindley, 1986).

Confidence, for both the clinician and the client, can have an effect on the outcome of therapy; therefore one has to balance the gains and losses for both parties produced by challenging 'adultism' and 'oppressiveness' in the way we have suggested here. As previously mentioned, a useful system to work with is the assertiveness-training one. This provides a framework based on self-respect and human rights, stressing mutuality. Asserting oneself is seen, not as winning at all costs, but as insisting upon one's right to be heard and to be reckoned with and according the same right to others, tiresome and inconvenient though this may prove!

KNOWLEDGE AND BELIEF CONCERNING LEARNING
AND BEHAVIOURAL CHANGE

Methods of education and therapy reflect not only attitudes but psychological theory and research. In setting out to equip people for life or to alter and improve their communicative behaviour one reveals the priorities one holds, one's beliefs concerning human beings and the way they learn and change. As Johnston (1983) pointed out, these constitute one's theories. Some favour purely cognitive approaches, others advocate a 'holistic' (body, mind and spirit) approach, some believe that the emotional life supercedes or motivates all learning and others again emphasize the importance of exploratory or physically active learning. Responsibility and decision making too are handled differently by individual therapists and educators, some preferring to share these with the pupil, student or client and others taking them mostly upon themselves while casting the learner in a more passive role. It is not possible to claim that one approach is superior in cases of communicative difficulty, since research findings do not yet enable us to do so.

The learning theory embraced, whether consciously or unconsciously, will affect treatment, especially if it has been imperfectly understood or adopted in an automatized and inflexible manner. Fey (1986) explains four psychological theories and their relationships to speech therapy at some length. It may be helpful to condense Fey's explorations here.

1. Operant Learning Theory (see behaviourism, above)
   Learning depends on the relationship between a stimulus, a response and the stimulus which follows the response (i.e. a reward or punishment). Therefore, sentences (and presumably other language structures) should be trainable by presenting an event or a picture and simultaneously presenting a sentence which describes it. The learner would be encouraged to imitate this verbal stimulus and subsequently be reinforced, either positively or negatively, for the performance. This theory underlies many of the procedures currently

in use in speech therapy clinics (Clinical Interaction; Chapter 3).

2. Social Learning Theory

Behaviour is indeed subject to external control but internal processes interact with the external ones in a complex fashion. Attention and motivation are important factors. The learner is still presented with target utterances and reinforced for correct production but immediate imitation is not required, neither is complete or perfect reproduction expected. Care is taken to provide a congenial personal model from whom the learner is expected to derive suitable utterances for a variety of circumstances. Many clinicians who regard operant learning theory as over-simple for language teaching have adopted this variation.

3. The Interactionist Viewpoint

Language is a complex system involving at least three elements: content, form and use. These knowledge bases interact with one another (Bloom and Lahey, 1978). Knowledge in each of these areas is constantly undergoing change and development as a result of the learner's interaction with the world. External factors influence rather than control learning, which proceeds according to the learner's existing knowledge and personal interest. Since what the learner will wish to express is not completely predictable, item learning/teaching cannot supply all his or her language needs. What is needed is encouragement to construct utterances (albeit imperfectly) on the basis of what is already known. The facilitative manipulation of the learner's environment should allow the necessary inductions to be made for relating language content, form and use. This will be more successful than attempting to teach the relations directly.

Clinicians who accept this viewpoint often hedge their bets by conducting some direct or indirect facilitative therapy (e.g. playing with a child and encouraging parents to do likewise) but at a different time clearly modelling or training target utterances or acceptable social behaviours. There is nothing to lose by this practice unless it interferes with the natural active involvement of the learner during facilitative time. Unfortunately, it is frequently allowed to do so. Once having assumed a passive role, clients all too often retain it and may be subtly encouraged to do so by the clinician's attitude. Fey considers interactionist theory the most appropriate basis for language therapy. It is also the basis of pragmatic therapy.

4. The Innatist Theory

   Language (i.e. syntax) is an independent, rule-governed system which can be manipulated by human beings in a variety of contexts (Chomsky, 1965). Learning the rules of the language system (i.e. how to transform meanings into a variety of surface forms) appears to be easy because humans are pre-programmed to do so. From this point Fey suggests that an unwarranted assumption has been made by clinicians. This is that when communicative skill fails to develop or is lost, clients should be taught syntactic categories, phrase structure and even transformational rules. A more promising clinical adaptation of Chomsky's work would be to view the client as one who actively, though usually unconsciously, builds linguistic competence by absorbing meanings and inducing rules for their expression in the normal pre-programmed fashion, but who perhaps requires longer exposure, to clearer language data than other learners in order to do so. A client might also require assistance in converting competence to performance but this would be given in realistic social situations and through the experience of assisted, confidence-building interactions rather than through syntactically based exercises. In this way, a realistic awareness of the size and complexity of the language learning task would be retained together with the awareness that step by step teaching of syntax is likely to have limited effect. Only when more naturalistic approaches to language facilitation are not proving satisfactory would attempts be made to provide language instruction by more formal methods. Even in these circumstances we would argue that teaching or encouraging the client to communicate and to attend to signals in a variety of modalities should be seen as of equal importance to language teaching.

IMPAIRED PERFORMANCE VS. DISABILITY

In Chapter 5 we discussed the importance of differentiating between behaviour and knowledge. This differentiation needs to be made in all instances of communicative difficulty. If phonology is disordered, what the listener hears is unexpected but the possible reasons why the client is speaking in this unexpected way are many and varied. Not all of the reasons involve a disability in phonological learning or processing. A similar situation exists with regard to disordered syntax. Not all disordered articulation arises from articulatory disability (a person may be careless or have uncomfortable teeth or may even be imitating or acting). If clinicians' minds are clear on this point, they can begin to differentiate between the client who is struggling with a disability and one who possesses the necessary abilities but requires help in mobilizing and utilizing these. Not only will treatment techniques differ in the two cases but also the therapist's expectations and the advice given to the client, their family and their associates will be different. Bridging the gap between competence and performance is a skilled therapeutic activity, yet a misconception exists that true therapeutic success involves only the teaching of new material. It can be hypothesized, on the contrary, that over-zealous attempts to instil new knowledge and behaviours results only in limited gains, whereas the mobilization of existing knowledge and ability results not only in short-term benefit to the individual but in longer term improvement in the ability to acquire new information and skill. Research has hardly begun to address the relationship of underlying competence and surface performance in communicative disability.

GENERALIZATION

Given a clear understanding of the importance of differentiating impaired pragmatic performance from pragmatic disability, it is possible to arrive at clinical aims and methods which maximize any abilities which the client does possess, concurrently with remediating deficits, where possible, and teaching compensatory strategies where necessary (Chapter

3). For too long some psychologists and speech clinicians concentrated upon teaching skills, behaviours and knowledge of language to a passive client, leaving the question of generalization to be dealt with at a later stage, only to discover that generalization presented a formidable challenge at a time when treatment had been assumed to be almost complete (Leonard, 1981). Suggestions for meeting this challenge will be found in many post-Leonard texts, in more detail than can be provided here. Hughes (1985), for example, recommends choosing functional targets; teaching enough examples; choosing the best examples; teaching several examples simultaneously; teaching 'loosely'; varying the antecedents; varying the consequences; programming the natural environment and teaching self-monitoring. Leith (1984) devotes a chapter to the topic of generalization, emphasizing the importance of clients' attitudes, emotions and motivation. He recommends extending the clinical process to clients' external environments and making considerable use of 'significant others' as helpers.

Similarly, Rosenbek, La Pointe and Wertz (1989) advise clinicians to prepare for generalization during the treatment of aphasia rather than praying for it once treatment has been completed. They stress that generalization can never be guaranteed but consider that it is made more likely by exposing patients to sufficient repetition. 'Ten repetitions are usually too few and several hundred may be just right' (p. 138). Similarly, it is suggested that as many as, say, a hundred items should be presented in any given category (e.g. foods, animals, plants). Clients should be taught to use self-generated cues and encouraged to become as independent as possible by learning 'to use their treated responses when they want to rather than when their clinicians want them to' (p. 138). Further recommendations include involving the patient and family in treatment and its planning, extending treatment outside the clinic by means of assignments and activities and teaching general activities such as relaxation together with specific items and skills.

Our clinical experience suggests that one of the most effective measures for insuring generalization is to share responsibility with clients and to encourage the performance of spontaneous communicative acts in a manner which actively involves them and engages their full attention. Together with the key policy of following their cues, so as to teach matters which relate directly to their personal lives, this seems to result in the reduction of any division between lessons and life. In order to make further progress in the understanding of how to promote generalization, there is an urgent need to research these methods, and the very least that clinicians who feel drawn to them should be prepared to do is to keep the kind of treatment records that would assist such research. That is to say, that clients' pre- and post-treatment performance should be assessed and described in social as well as linguistic terms, possibly making use of some of the assessment materials mentioned in Chapter 6. The methods of treatment used should be described in some detail, though not necessarily at every session. If clinicians who do not wish to engage in research were to make such data available, it would provide valuable background information for the rigorous investigation of interactive methods. At present, inadequate clinical approaches can usually be justified, if challenged, by pointing out that some progress is being made, even though little social improvement is evident.

HIGH-QUALITY INTERACTIONS

It can be hypothesized that faster and more easily generalized learning will take place when the client is exposed to at least some high-quality interactive experiences. What high-quality interaction entails could be explored in relation to one's own experiences, by identifying the relationships and situations which enable one to experience the most satisfying communication. What are their characteristics? What is the interaction like? Try to describe it and to focus upon the features which contribute toward your satisfaction. Here is an example:

> I communicate well with a speech therapy colleague whom I have known for a long time, especially when we are alone and talking about work. Things go better if we are not tired or rushed and if neither of us wishes to

enforce a particular view of the matter under discussion. She is a good person to talk to because:

1. She listens carefully to me, leaves space for me, takes me seriously and doesn't question my credentials.
2. She tells me plainly what she thinks and doesn't pretend to thoughts and feelings that she does not demonstrate to be genuine.
3. When we interrupt one another, this gets sorted out amicably. The same is true if one of us wants to change the topic or to be silent for a while.
4. She talks about things which interest me and is interested in matters which I want to raise.
5. We don't have to be serious all the time and I can let her know my true feelings, not always positive or respectable ones.
6. She follows through on matters that we have discussed.
7. She surprises me.
8. She gives me information that is really useful both professionally and personally.
9. If we have a misunderstanding we can repair it.
10. We apologise if we upset one another.
11. When I am not sure how to express myself she works with me on the idea until it is clear, rather than imposing one of her own or hurrying the interaction.
12. Sometimes we are able to guess at one another's thoughts, with rather little in the way of language to cue us in.

Creating a personal example in this way enables one to see ideal communication more clearly than, for instance, Grice's conversational maxims do (Chapters 1 and 4). In the same way one can explore unsatisfactory interactions within one's own personal experience (e.g. 'She makes me feel I have no valid contribution to make; she is not interested in what I have to say. She doesn't listen or listens selectively . . .'). Studying such familiar experiences highlights the negotiated nature of relationships and the sharing of responsibility for success and failure.

Having examined personal experiences in this way we are then in a strong position to evaluate the interactive experiences available to the client. Has the client in hospital

a visitor to hold hands with? Has the young child a congenial playmate? The value of such relationships needs to
be appreciated by those involved with the client, so that
they will be developed and not inadvertently discouraged,
because the importance of relationships is sometimes under-
estimated by clients' families.

If no high-quality interaction is available, it is essential
to provide some. This can be done by a clinician, who will
need to be skilled in responding to minimal signals from
the client and building them gradually and enjoyably into
interactive skills. Another part of the clinician's role has
long been recognized as being 'indirect'. This work is concerned with adjusting clients' environments so that they
become more facilitative. Relatives can be encouraged to
end a client's social isolation, despite the difficulties or perhaps embarrassment of doing so. They can also be shown
effective methods of helping the client to communicate.
This is not to state that families cause communication problems unilaterally; they may however perpetuate them in
some cases (cf. Fey 1986, Leonard 1987, Puckering and
Rutter, 1987; see also Chapter 5). Nurses, teachers and
speech-language clinicians themselves also need to ensure
that they are familiar with a suitable range of communicatively facilitative behaviours and are not unwittingly
restricting clients' development or recovery. It could be
suggested that only people who have experienced satisfying, empathic interactions will be motivated to improve
their interactive behaviour. Such experiences should also
provide them with an example of how to relate to another
human being enjoyably and how to take the perspective
of others.

'TOP-DOWN VS. BOTTOM-UP' APPROACHES

'Top-down' and 'bottom-up' refer to concepts which have
been familiar for many years in the field of deaf education.
Some teachers attempt to teach the components of speech
and language in a series of small steps, beginning with the
linguistically 'simplest' (e.g. phonemes, words, phrases,
sentences). This was known at one time as 'analytic method'
and could be seen as a 'bottom-up' approach. Other teachers

maintain that learning is facilitated by the presentation of meaningful chunks of language which are only later split into their component parts in order to highlight and improve specific details. This was known as 'synthetic method' and can be seen as 'top-down' teaching. A further illustration can be constructed by imagining inexperienced musicians preparing to play an elaborate composition. Some conductors might commence by perfecting certain very small sections, particular notes, entrances and solo passages (i.e. bottom-up). Others, thinking that the performers would find this more meaningful, might expect to study the piece as a whole or to attempt run-throughs of quite large sections before perfecting details (i.e. top-down). The notion here is that a task which holds interest and meaning is motivating despite its apparent difficulty.

Speech-language clinicians tend to work within the 'bottom-up' model because they know that linguistically complex structures present difficulty to clients. They are also used to thinking in terms of hierarchies of linguistic structures where more complex structures are composed of simpler ones. Complexity and simplicity would be determined in relation to the number of words per utterance and in relation to the number of embedded clauses. Communicative activity however can be thought of as having a different structure in which complex linking of ideas may have simple linguistic correlates. For instance, a child uttering 'horsie gen' appears linguistically unsophisticated but must have been able to connect knowledge of the world, desire for the reoccurrence of the horse, pragmatic knowledge including knowledge of intonation and gesture with intention and linguistic knowledge. A person uttering a linguistically more elaborate version of the same request ('Please I would love to have the horse again if you don't mind.') would have performed the same underlying processes. The 'top-down' model of therapy works with the notion that human beings are capable of complex communicative processing without necessarily possessing all the linguistic prerequisites for complex performance. It is also based on the supposition that interest in and commitment to the meaning of an exchange will provide motivation for improving some of its component parts. As such it will employ conversation, narrative, activity, poetry, song and play of various kinds (for both children and adults) in combination with corrective exercises to produce improvements in communicative performance. Even clinicians' silence may be valuable in the top-down approach in order to provide space for meaning-driven contributions from actively involved clients.

PRINCIPLES FOR PRAGMATICS-BASED THERAPY

By coalescing a summary of the treatment implications of previous chapters with the summary of the general issues discussed in the current chapter, we are now able to arrive at a set of general principles for pragmatics-based therapy. Since the principles are derived from the fairly detailed and explicit arguments already put forward, it should be possible for others to design well-reasoned treatment plans and research programmes, depending on which of our suppositions individuals find interesting.

1. Changing what a person knows, thinks and feels will be as influential in improving that person's communicative success as attempting to change that person's behaviour.
2. Personally relevant goals will attract the client's full attention and co-operation. Clients learn for their own purposes and integrate what is learnt for the same reason.
3. Poor performance does not necessarily indicate poor ability. Confidence is crucial. Enhancing confidence is part of the clinician's role. Clients who are allowed and encouraged to perform voluntary speech acts gain confidence. Stereotyped expectations, on the other hand, can lead to malfunctioning clients.
4. If language learning is functionally driven (i.e. communication motivates learning) interactive therapy and improvements in pragmatic skill should produce improvement in other linguistic capabilities.
5. An important distinction exists between the surface manifestations of problems and their underlying causes. Either or both may be treated.

6. Much of the knowledge clients require may be unconscious and may therefore be difficult to acquire through direct instruction. Enhancing metapragmatic awareness, on the other hand, may be helpful.
7. Narrative skill may be crucial to discourse development and to acquisition of and maintenance of other components of communicative ability.
8. Deterioration of pragmatic behaviours due to environmental influences is likely to be reversible but may lead to reduced pragmatic competence in some circumstances.
9. Problems of processing language at the normal speed may be especially destructive to pragmatic performance and must be compensated for.
10. Problems of not only lexical and syntactic comprehension but also pragmatic comprehension merit careful attention. Such problems may concern non-verbal communication, inference and evaluation. In other words, pragmatic comprehension involves retaining, connecting and interpreting both denotative and connotative meanings however these are expressed.
11. Assessment for intervention demands that the goals most likely to be achieved (which are not necessarily developmentally early ones) should be identified and given priority in treatment. These should be followed by the goals most closely related to improvements in communicative effectiveness (e.g. intelligibility or the ability to ask questions or perform useful speech acts). Other theoretically appropriate goals should be introduced only when clients can be motivated toward them.
12. The notions of pragmatic 'knowing that' and pragmatic 'knowing how' (Chapter 5) provide indications as to what a client may need to know in order to have a chance of functioning in communication. Linking pragmatic knowledge to severity of disturbance (Chapter 5) provides further guidance as to which aspects of one's pragmatic problem may require more urgent attention. Moreover, research into treatment effectiveness could be based on hypotheses concerning underlying pragmatic knowledge.
13. In treatment (and assessment) the value of positive communication strategies should be borne in mind.

The use of apparently inappropriate communicative behaviour may constitute an achievement strategy (Chapter 3).

SUMMARY

In this chapter it is suggested that carefully structured treatment within which the client is free to initiate and use responses which serve as further initiations can also include some correction and specific instruction. The essential point about pragmatics-based therapy is that the client is not cast in a passive role, but is helped to use communicative behaviour for his or her own purposes. It is claimed that this type of therapy may accelerate clients' progress and that its effectiveness needs to be researched as a matter of urgency. Such research needs to take into account the ways in which clinicians' views and beliefs concerning social roles and learning mechanisms are reflected in the type of therapy offered to poorly communicating clients.

Our fundamental hypothesis is that since communicative performance demands the integration of complex knowledge and a variety of skills, the client's confidence to experiment with imperfect abilities is crucial to the acquisition and mobilization of communicative competence. The need for the client to be defensive should not arise in situations designed to be therapeutic.

In the next chapter four young people with communication problems are presented as examples of the application of pragmatics-based therapy.

Chapter 8

Clinical examples

The following clinical examples are intended to provide data concerning the interactive style employed in pragmatics-based therapy. This style contrasts with the more directive approaches described by Letts (1985, 1989), Panagos, Bobkoff and Scott (1986) and Ripich and Panagos (1985) (Chapter 3). It is neither completely permissive nor coercive but tries to maintain an equilibrium. While the therapist may still be asking rather more questions than would be recommended for maximally facilitative interaction, they were questions to which she did not yet know the answers. The examples indicate that the improvements which occurred are no worse, and may possibly be better, than those normally expected.

Much abbreviated case histories of four children, two with severe and two with moderate communicative difficulties, will be presented. Samples of communicative behaviour and some comment as to how these people and their problems can be viewed in the light of previous sections will be provided. Each of the children was encouraged to perform a variety of speech acts and to acquire an interest in imaginative play and story books. Care was taken to foster lexical acquisition, intelligibility, memory and narrative skill. In order to provide opportunities for the child to initiate, the adult tries to avoid claiming all the available communicative space. Further case information can be provided on request although identities have been protected by altering the children's names and some other details. Prosodic information is not included here, but has been considered in interpreting the data.

SIMON

Simon currently attends his local secondary (comprehensive) school, where he is supported by Special Needs staff and appears to be learning a reasonable amount and to be making some social contact with other students. He shines at computer tasks. He appears contented despite the fact that his communicative difficulties were at one time so severe that he was perceived by various professionals as suffering from brain damage, extreme distress, 'semantic-pragmatic disorder', language disorder or Asperger's Syndrome. Timely attention to the aspects of his problem which hindered communicative functioning would have been more helpful than these conflicting diagnoses.

Before entering the current school, Simon was placed in a special school for children with learning disability. He and his family resented the placement and persuaded the local authority to return him to the main stream.

Simon first became known to the authors on entering junior school at the age of 10 having moved from another area. It transpired that his early life had included referral to a Department of Child and Family Psychiatry, for communicative and developmental difficulties, including toilet training problems. Evidence from that period is sketchy but on closing the case when Simon was aged 4;9 the consultant psychiatrist commented 'The child is now dry by day; parents are pleased with progress; vocabulary is coming on fast; the child is bright and alert, enjoys school, likes his teacher and has some friends.' It was also stated that he 'played constructively with toy materials' and that 'some articulatory defect is present but improving'. However, nine months later the consultant replied to a letter from the Clinical Medical Officer at the Central School Clinic thus: 'I was interested to read your account of Simon's behaviour at school. . . . I see that I specifically mentioned the reasonable quality of Simon's expressive speech (in my previous letter) therefore the comment of Simon's class teacher is apposite (relevant) and I am wondering whether the lad is in any way "switching off" '. Clearly the class teacher had found communicative difficulties.

Simon's pronunciation appears to have been generally

intelligible, which may account for the fact that it was not until the age of 7;3 that he was referred by his school and an Educational Psychologist for speech therapy. At that time both expressive language and comprehension were assessed, by a number of methods, as delayed by approximately three years and six months. Due to the parents' reluctance to accept the need for therapy and to the pressure of other cases, he was then placed on a waiting list 9–12 months long, though consultative help was provided by the speech therapist for the school. A year later the delay was measured as two years five months but regular therapy was again refused. The Educational Psychologist reported 'a mixture of problems; very poor language skills, developmental difficulties in visual motor skills; educational and social problems stemming from these; an unsettled domestic situation' but added, 'Despite these he has made some progress in his reading and social adjustment since entering junior school.' Another year later it was thought that Simon should be statemented as having special educational needs under the Education Act which had been passed three years previously. He subsequently moved into the Junior School where we encountered him. This school is one that has a commitment to children with special needs and has certain resources, facilities, experience and attitudes not widely available in 'normal schools'.

Simon, at the age of ten, was first observed by the current authors at this school, skirting the perimeter of the playground, looking at no one, taking no part in games and appearing pre-occupied and dejected. He did not respond to classroom events or to direct remarks, other than by occasional short utterances and fleeting eye contact. In one-to-one speech therapy he appeared anxious, looked downward, used flat intonation, gave minimal replies to questions, showed little curiosity or interest in activities and never initiated conversation. His behaviour gave rise to the suspicion that he had experienced some form of bullying or abuse, either from children or others. Since some speech therapy was available at school it was possible to offer treatment to Simon. While the parents gave only permission at the outset, his mother later became helpful and co-operative.

For the following reasons, it was decided that therapy based on pragmatic principles might prove more effective than speech-language instruction

1. This boy appeared to be unmotivated toward communication and to lack confidence in attempting speech.
2. Language development can be assumed to be motivated and facilitated by participation in communicative interaction.
3. Only one short period of speech-therapy contact time per week was available.
4. Short periods of communication-based therapy were thought to be more likely to provide information which could be utilized by relatives and members of staff who were in constant touch with Simon.
5. Some insight needed to be gained into Simon's interests, needs and abilities.

The initial aim of communication therapy was to convince Simon that interaction could be meaningful and that his limited language skills could be used to his advantage. To enlarge a linguistic repertoire that was unlikely to be used seemed purposeless.

Although he presented as an odd ten year old, it was felt that this child's comprehension and expressive language skills, which corresponded to those of a younger child, should at least have enabled him to function socially as a younger person would do. Therefore, a rather maternal style of interaction was adopted by therapist, teachers, and assistants. Utterances addressed to him were kept short, simple and concerned as far as possible with Simon's focus of attention. Only as he became more confident were utterances lengthened. If he did not seem able to respond they were rephrased and visual cues were provided. After three months of rather slow progress Simon was placed in class beside another child (Edward) with communication difficulties. Teachers felt that a friendship developed between the two which proved beneficial in both cases. The speech therapist had reservations about the quality of interaction taking place within this relationship, however a breakthrough seemed to occur in the second month, as the following extract from classroom observation notes makes clear:

"Edward was not apparently listening to teacher. Simon obviously was.

Simon said, quietly, 'I wish there was' when told that there would be no colouring.

Simon was vocalizing sensibly to self, while drawing and giving instructions to Edward.

Edward hindered him with comments such as 'It's a picture Simon, there's a picture' and did no drawing himself.

Simon muttered to therapist 'Edward says that windmill's small. It isn't, it's massive'. (The class had recently visited a windmill.)

Edward suggested that the height was about eight feet, ten feet, twenty, forty, eighty or sixty, but Simon stuck to a hundred feet saying that he counted as they climbed up. He commented that he had finished his picture and actually repeated the comment because I had not heard. Subsequent conversation about the trip was consistently satisfactory. Simon answered questions appropriately, though not quite directly

e.g. T. Did they actually grind up flour there?
  S. Everyone was buying flour, they (the flour bags) had a picture of a windmill on.

Simon and Therapist could not make sense of Edward's questions or statements and Simon appeared to lack the social skills to handle this problem.

No one else attempted to join the interaction."

After these observation notes had been circulated there was considerable discussion amongst staff. Clearly Simon could interact more effectively than had previously been thought, given an attentive listener (i.e. the speech therapist). Possibly the 'friendship' with Edward served the purpose of ending social isolation for them both and providing an experience of superiority for Simon, but it could not take the place of more intensive therapy for Edward or of high quality interaction for Simon. Now that the value of sensitive, responsive individual attention had been demonstrated, it was provided for him on a more regular basis by teachers and support staff. Although the adults' style remained maternal in some respects, it was felt by all staff, including the speech therapist, that exaggerated intonation would seem unduly patronising. However, hindsight inclines us to think that it should have been employed for two reasons. Firstly, it was noted much later that such emphasis greatly assisted Simon's comprehension and, secondly, his own intonation patterns remained abnormally flat, despite a little improvement when talking with peers.

Circumstances were such that an average of less than half-an-hour of direct speech therapy per week was available to this seriously disabled boy who still spoke rarely in school. During therapy sessions speed of utterance was reduced on the part of the therapist to assist Simon's comprehension. Careful attention was paid to his non-verbal signals. Intriguing objects such as sparklers, picture books, various spinning and jumping toys, pop-up books, 'pop' tapes, a kaleidoscope etc. were offered in an attempt to overcome passivity. Silence was employed deliberately so that ample opportunities for initiation were available to the less confident partner and silence was tolerated while he slowly formulated responses to questions. Sometimes this could take up to 14 seconds and it was necessary to check, intuitively or by direct enquiry, whether or not he had given up the attempt to reply. Teachers found information about this time-lag helpful. Care was taken to convince Simon that utterances were expected at all times to be meaningful and to relate to one another. This was done by means of arranging 'pay-off' for his utterances and gently insisting on follow-up for those of the therapist. The classroom examples had proved this to be possible but satisfying conversation was rare at that stage.

An example of 'pay-off' for communication follows. Groups of children were seen passing the window of the therapy room, therefore both Simon and the therapist rose to watch them rather than persisting with the task in hand. One of his rare initiations was triggered.

S. It's my class.
T. Where are they going?
S. Football. (Silence)
T. Do you want to go to football?
S. Yes. (Appears surprised)
T. Go on then. Come back here after football.

Simon maintained eye contact for some time, before leaving, changing and going to football. He returned with minimal prompting.

There are children for whom this type of negotiation of therapy time could be seen as unnecessarily indulgent, but for Simon it was a crucial part of communication therapy.

Another therapeutic measure was concerned with narrative skills. A vagueness had been observed in attention to visual or spoken narrative and this was thought to relate to lack of comprehension and difficulty in maintaining a coherent view of the action or significance of stories. Discussion of attractive picture books was therefore introduced and, again, there was gentle insistence upon the discourse features of the illustrations rather than their individual significance.

S. The rabbit's thin.
T. The rabbit's suddenly got much thinner. What happened?
S. Silence
T. Let's look back at the other pages. The boy sat on it, then, after that, the stuffing was coming out, then. . . .
S. The stuffing's on the floor.
T. Yes, that's why the rabbit looks so thin. The stuffing's not inside; it's on the floor.

At one stage Simon explained that he was unable to remember earlier events in narratives, and therefore some time was spent in improving either his ability to memorize or to recall or to trust himself to be able to do these things. One could never be quite sure which aspect of memory was crucial but an improvement took place and he began to behave as if the coherence of stories was more apparent to him than previously, as was the discourse significance of certain events within the stories. The following interruption initiated by Simon during casual discussion of a picture story was regarded as a significant landmark in his progress. He had remembered an observation previously made and connected it to the development of a story.

S. Look. There's that bit. (that we were talking about earlier)
T. Where?
S. There. Look.
T. Oh I see.
Oh, so they *were* telling him to get up then?
S. Yes they were.

By the time he left junior school at age 12 Simon was beginning to be interested in and tolerant of language correction and, as he talked more freely, his language problems became more apparent. It was also discovered that he often made serious mistakes in interpreting facial expression, both in life and in picture books. This was thought to be connected with his own poor use of facial expression. Similar two-way difficulties have been reported in people suffering from right hemisphere damage and from Parkinsonism (Scott; Caird and Williams 1985; Code 1987). It is not known whether he could have been taught to interpret facial expression more accurately.

The teacher's comment, after writing her formal report on transfer from junior to senior school, was significant. 'Well, he's certainly not the "idiot-boy" he once was (seemed to be), but whether he's learnt a lot or just got a lot more confident is anybody's guess.'

Chronological data

Some chronological data will now be provided which illustrates the changes that were taking place in Simon's communicative behaviour, between entry to the special unit at junior school, at which time he spoke very little, and entry to senior school, at which time he could hold a reasonable conversation.

Year 1. December Aged 10; Conversation about Toys:
T. Do you know what these two are?
S. No.

T. See if you can find out what it does.
S. Goes to bits.
T. Does it?
S. Goes to bits.
T. I see, you show me.
S. It goes like that. It moves.
T. And how do you make it do that?
S. Cos it stands in there.
T. So what do you have to do to make it do that?
S. Spring.
T. It's on a spring is it?
S. Yes.
T. How do you make it speed around?
S. Press on . . . goes in the air.
T. That's far enough I think.

Year 2. January Narration with picture book. Simon speaks as he turns the pages.

1. John lived with his . . . (silence).
2. A boy's holding a sheep and there's a dog barking.
3. The boy's giving the horse a eat and the boy's holding the horse.
4. The man's fishing.
5. A dog's barking.
6. There's a stream there, some horses near the mountain.
7. The boy's holding a hat (saddle) and there's all mans going round sheep. All the mans are shouting.
8. A boy's going to bed.
9. The boy's shouting at the people.
10. The people said the people want to go to bed.
11. The horses are going somewhere.
12. The people saw some sheep.
13. They saw a hill, saw a rock, dogs are running, there's horse at top of the hill.
14. The people have got swords (sticks).
15. The people got stuck in the snow.
(T. What do you think about it? Do you like it?
S. Yes. (The story is now beginning to interest him.)
16. The people got lost in the snow.
17. The boy was near the dog.
18. The boy was going up that mountain.

19. The boy's riding the horse.
20. They saw a sheep stuck.
21. The boy was getting the sheep.
22. The boy was going up the mountain.
23. The dog was walking along the snow.
24. The boy was asleep.
25. The dog went at the door.
(One would not realize from these statements that the boy had become trapped on the ledge with the sheep he had been attempting to rescue or that the dog had therefore gone to seek help.)
26. The people were riding in the snow.
    (Coming to the rescue.)
27. They're getting a rope for the boy.
28. They were picking the sheep up.
29. They pulled the boy up.
30. And they're walking up along the snow.
31. The sheep walk along the mountain.
32. The boy went to bed.

The same story is now re-told, at the same session, without looking at the book.

S. The people were walking on the snow. They walked on the mountain. All the people went up the mountain.

The story was then re-read by Simon whose mechanical reading was developing rapidly. He also looked at the pictures. This is his subsequent re-telling without looking at the book.

S. He went fishing. The boy went to bed. The people saw some sheep. The dog went up.

Loss of interest could well have explained the poor performance but further discussion revealed that this was not the case. Simon's explanation was that he found it difficult to remember the story without the pictures. This was not surprising since no narrative thread seemed to exist for him.

Year 2. May Extract from conversation between Simon and the Therapist

T. . . . and my keys were inside the house but the door was shut. It was a terrible nuisance.

S. My Mum done that at the keys one time and what you
   have to do is you have to chuck something into the
   window and get in.

However, Simon could not make any attempt to answer
hypothetical questions of the type 'What should I do
if . . . ?'

Year 2. July Reporting a playground incident.
T. Who was in trouble?
S. Ian and he throwed the hard ball and he hit the window and he smashed the window and he brokened it.
   He was in the playground and he throwed the hard
   balled and Mrs (Mr) Jones told our class about it. He
   took the ball off Ian and he told him off.

The fact that this is much improved reporting, was perceived as outweighing the need for grammatical correction.

Year 2. September Simon is being encouraged to outline
his aims for the new school year.
T. I'd like to write down what you would like to learn.
S. Yes.
T. OK. Now we've got to think about what you'd like to
   do for this term. How you getting on (um) in the
   playground? Have you got friends?
S. No.
T. Not yet?
   What about football. How's that going?
S. Can't play.
T. Why?
S. Cos I can't kick.
   Well can't even kick, can't even get the ball.
T. But you like football, don't you?
S. Yes but I can't even get the ball at all. It's too difficult
   to get a kick.
T. How much practice do you get Simon?
S. –
T. Do you get a chance to play on your own to practise?
   Do you know what I mean practise?
S. Yes. Means you gonna try and see how good you are
   (be) for the . . .
T. Yes. That's right (It wasn't really). Do you get a chance
   to do that?

S. (8 second pause) No
T. Do you want – shall I put that on my list of things that you want to do?
S. Yes.
T. You, that you want to learn, I'm going to make a list of things you want to learn. Can you see a pencil?
S. There.
T. Right, Simon wants to learn better kicking.
S. Yes.
T. Making friends?
S. Yes.
T. What sort of things does Mrs M teach you?
S. Maths, English, jotter.
T. What's that? Don't understand, say it again.
S. Jotter.
T. What is it? What could that be?
   Jotter (puzzled).
S. Yes. It's where you put words and that.
T. Oh. Is it spelt like that?
S. Yes.
T. Ah. Jotter. It's where you jot down words that fit into things. That's where you got that 'undulation' one to do?
S. Yes.
T. Yes. Yes.
   Anything else you would specially like to learn?
S. Topic, science. Think that's about. . . .
T. Think that's about it?
S. Yes.
T. OK. So now we know what we're doing.

Year 2: October Therapist's classroom observation notes.
It is the type of lesson (sewing) in which children are expected to chat quietly. Simon appears to understand this. He listens to others as well as speaking to them, still too loudly. Someone eventually says 'Shut up Simon'. He replies 'What can I do if I can't do it (sew) though?' Someone says 'Ask Mrs F'. He joins her queue but goes back to place and asks others to help him find a lost needle but they tire of this so he uses exaggerated searching behaviour to gain teacher's attention. Concentration

is good, on the whole, but he worries and distracts himself and others by remarks such as 'I can't do it; it's too titchy; all it's doing is just making holes' etc. When the other children move away he talks more. When I went to help him he used the following with reasonable intonation 'Look, if you watch this, it gets all tangled up.' 'I can't do it.' 'How come there's no sewing going on?' (The thread had pulled through but when I tied a knot in it he thought that was intended to prevent the tangling rather than the pulling through.) Child says 'Have you got the hang of it now?' Simon replies 'I've got the hang of it, I'm getting the hang of it.' Secures help when the cotton runs out but keeps repeating 'I don't know how I got short of cotton.' The boy detailed to help him says 'There's a good boy (!) That's better stitching than me, I'm serious.' Simon asks questions but when shown what to do says 'Just *tell* me.' Later he says 'This is the first time I've sewn.'

Year 2. December Simon is dictating a story to the Therapist. 'When we went down the hillside it was rather soggy and there was a lake in the middle of the landscape. Then, then when we went down the landscape there were people playing cricket in the sun . . . then we were sledging through the woods, then we saw like a bridge, then, then we just stopped to look at it. Then there was water in the way splashing and splashing. Then there was all rocks and minerals and trees . . . then when we went on the bridge it was going to start to snap. . . . Then when we ran down on the bridge we saw some and saw some ice all floating on the water, then we were going to rush, thought it was going to break and we had to go back as soon as possible.' (Beyond this point the story became less coherent.)

Year 3. March Dictated story
'We are going take some photos down the valley, then we walk across and see a house. It was all like all straw and all breaking. The wood was all snapping off at the top. We are going to stay until night. Then in the afternoon it was going to start to rain so we might as well stay in 'til it brighten up. Then for a bit we saw it getting darker. The rain it was really slushing it out. Then it was starting to

all flood in the house and we were going up after and it was breaking. Then there was all wood flying off the top. We were frightened.' (This is approximately half the story, which was one of many very similar ones connected to real life events.)

Year 3. May Simon initiates and comments more frequently.
S. (On meeting Therapist outside classroom)
   There's a mistake on page 43. It doesn't make sense.
   You came to see my mum. Was it you?
   Did you talk to my rabbit?
   Did you see my computer?

By now Simon's speed of utterance and intonation had improved somewhat and facial expression was more lively. Poverty of vocabulary was apparent but he accepted new words eagerly and used them. Simon's vocabulary test scores improved dramatically at this stage. He accepted and used grammatical corrections but continued to experience difficulty in estimating what his listeners already knew and what they needed to be told. He also still had difficulty with problems such as 'If John hurt himself what could you do?' with the exception of those he had personally experienced.

Year 4. November Aged 13; Conversation with one of the authors
L. That's a good story, but I find it quite difficult to understand. Why d'you think I find it difficult to understand?
S. I don't know.
L. Is it because I have never seen it (a film)?
S. No.
L. No? D'you think I should understand it from this?
S. Yes.
L. Um 'cause I'm not always sure what "they" . . . cos you say they did something and they did something' I'm not always sure what they refer to. Cos I don't know.
S. Yes.
L. I haven't seen the film.
   D'you understand what I'm saying?

S. Yes.

L. So, how d'you think you could make it sometimes more understandable?

S. (5 seconds) Don't know.

L. Maybe instead of saying *'they* did something and *they* did such and such' you could say who they are.

S. The people?

L. Is it all about the people, is it?

S. Yes.

L. The people did . . . Is it a group of people?

S. Yes.

L. Um er OK. How about the end?
Is that 'soldiers'?

S. Guarding.

L. Guarding. So he cut the rope?

S. Yes.

L. Who is he?

S. Indiana Jones.

L. Oh Indiana Jones?
Well you didn't say, did ya?

S. (laughing) What?

L. You didn't say Indiana Jones, did you?

S. At the start of it?

L. Where?

S. You mean should've it been mentioned?

L. Yeah. Don't you think?

S. Think it should be all mentioned all in the story as well?

L. Well it should have been said in the beginning cos I didn't know this was about Indiana Jones, cos I haven't seen the film have I?

S. No.

L. Cos otherwise I didn't know who he was.

In summary

1. There seems little doubt that communication therapy should have been available to this family at an early stage; ideally when Simon was aged 2;6–3;0 or when his mother first expressed concern.

2. Such therapy ought to have incorporated or proceeded in parallel with family counselling.

3. Such therapy ought to have covered pragmatic, linguistic and articulatory abilities and should have been available on an intensive basis.
4. Given the serious proportions which the problems had been allowed to reach, placement in a special teaching facility was helpful.
5. Pragmatic assessments were helpful to therapists and teachers but ought to have been carried out in a variety of settings, including the home, in order to determine whether the problem lay in the area of ability or confidence. Time should have been available for this purpose.
6. Close co-operation between educational psychologist, teaching-support staff and the speech therapist was beneficial, especially since video equipment was available and professionals were able to observe one another's work and Simon's response.
7. Speech therapy should have remained available with language as a priority, once Simon entered main stream senior school. This was not the case.
8. The question of whether placement in a language unit, language school, psychiatric unit or psychotherapy programme ought to have been offered to Simon and his parents at any stage remains open. Clearly he ought not to have been allowed to get into such difficulty after initially receiving attention for developmental problems.
9. Finally, it is salutary to note that Simon did not once speak to the taxi-driver who took him to and from school for three years. There was much that we should have taught him and did not.

JOHN AND DAVID

It is not uncommon for twins to develop a private language and to be slow to adapt to the language of their community. In John and David's case, several additional factors accounted for their referral to speech therapy, at age three, with good non-verbal communication but with spoken language that was sparse and intelligible only to their mother and the other twin. These factors included tongue-tie (John); hearing loss (both boys); enlarged tonsils and adenoids (both); stressed and hospitalized mother; new baby and suspected general language disability (David). It is our contention that disability is indicated, not by the type of language produced but by the child's difficulty in making use of cues and in understanding, retaining, recalling and using linguistic information. John was able to benefit from therapy more rapidly than David and was therefore regarded as having superior language skills to his brother. Attention was given by the speech therapist and students concerned to all the factors mentioned above in addition to articulation, auditory perception and memory, phonetic inventory/repertoire, phonology (the sound system), vocabulary, syntax (grammar), motivation, emotional well-being and communicative confidence. The multi-faced development of communicative competence was thus facilitated and the twins entered main stream school without serious difficulty. By the age of seven they passed for non-speech-handicapped children who displayed minor abnormalities of pronunciation and in David's case, some slowness in coping with classroom 'language work'. Throughout their period of regular attendance at speech therapy clinic they were expected to initiate as well as respond to conversational topics. They were also exposed to long stretches of language data in the form of stories, songs and rhymes and were expected to produce these themselves. Some would argue that the language samples which follow indicate the need to stop these children talking, and thus practising errors, until such time as they have been taught the correct forms to use. While developing language children experiment and constantly modify their productions so as to bring them into line with those of people around them. Children who have received excessive correction and those whose production of language has been inhibited in order to await the acquisition of skills appear to experiment less, take time to regain fluent production and, in the worst cases, never attain full communicative competence. Neglecting to foster such experimentation during the process of teaching specific skills might be said to constitute dereliction of duty towards the child just as neglecting to teach specific skills would do.

Chronological data

The samples that follow represent first the four-year-old twins' narration of the Shirley Hughes picture story 'Up and Up', in which a girl receives and eats a magic Easter egg which, to the consternation of others, enables her to fly (Hughes 1981). The picture book is used to assist these narrations.

John 4;6
Once upon a time there was girl, she seed bird and she gonned out. And she see all the birds and she tripped over rock and banged herself on his head. And he makes wings and his paints the wings black and he cuts wings out and puts them on. And he jumps with them on and the (sic) goes on ladder and he jumps and banged hiself again. And he blows up balloon and just blow up another one. And he blows and he puts strings. And he goes outside and he goes up and the stick burst it. And he goes inside and knock on a door. And he, um her, goes off tree, flies away. He runs after and he knock all vegetables off. And children in school see her and he looks out window and school children run away. And he makes patterns. And he goes in the big balloon and he going catcher her and she's going up and girl went on there. (On the television aerial) (Long unintelligible utterance) And inside house the television gone wrong and he banged it and it works. And he flies up, he flies away, he bursts it balloon. And girl stopped flying and she had dinner.

David 4;6
Little girl watching birds. Watched all birds and watched birds and tripped over banged i head and stars come, starts to cry. Colour wings and paper and cut them out. Climb up ladders and jumped out and banged bottom. Blow up balloons and put string on and go outside and fly and tree bust them. And (unintelligible) and postman bring (unintelligible) and little girl open it and cut the string and little girl got outside. Easter egg and girl inside it and started flying. It magic Easter egg and go up roof,

go on roof and walk on roof and upside down on wall (ceiling). Go over tea (tea-table) and fly outside and go be people waiting bus stop and fly past some more people try to catch her. And man looking telescope and man . . . and fly more peoples try catch her tree fly up girl and by a cart and try catch her up. His school or in window and teacher point and one one looking out and girl was looking in window. And saw out, look there is a girl (exhausted). Broken wire and television got worse and (unintelligible) and burst balloon and it fell down and her fly back and shake her hand and mummy kiss her (and daddy were happy (after prompting) and had egg.

The next sample involves only one twin but represents the typical conversational style of both at that stage of development. It is followed by a brief conversation recorded almost two years later.

6 years 5 months, David speaks to therapist who limits the length of her own utterances.

T. I think you said 'space ship' better than you did last week.
 I think the way you told the story was smashing. Why were you so tired this morning? You looked all sleepified.
D. I know. Cos I'd been to Blackpool last night.
T. Oh I see.
D. And I came back twe – twelve o'clock.
T. Oh no wonder you're half asleep.
D. I been and I was, my bed time was at nine o'clock, spose to go in at nine o'clock.
T. I see.
D. Daddy was, Daddy couldn't get awake. So tired when he drive all away. Mummy drive only to a garage. When Daddy drive all a way and drive back.
T. Goodness me.
D. Yes.
T. Was it good? Was it worth going?
D. (Pause) Ah, it was! That were (dialectal) a lot of fun. I got all soakid.
T. Did you?

D. Yeah. You come up this ride, you slide down, when you smashed, when you're going water go smashed (splashed) you get wet.

T. Really? I love those. Have you ever been on a water-shoot?

D. (Minimal response).

T. They're marvellous, aren't they?

D. Mm. And I was already wet while it was raining.

T. You were already wet so you didn't care if you got a bit wetter?

D. When (it or I) came out we dried up.

T. You got dry cos it was fairly warm?

D. Mm. Sun came out. When we going home it get raining again. I got wet again.

T. Oh dear. But it was a really good trip?

D. (Nods).

T. Well that's great.

D. Got these um, we had um, got loads of 1 ps, right? You put them. You got a thing and you put 1p in and it slides down and you have it, to and, push it and these things push it the money out and when it lands on the top of something you can't win it!

In the final sample both twins talk briefly to the therapist.

7;6 John and David

T.   How's Jim getting on?

D.   He's getting on fine.

J.   Yes. He's going to start school on a little while.

D.   Well he's going to. After Christmas he going to start school.

J.   He goes to play school on Thursday and Friday.

T.   He seems really happy.

D.   Doesn't when he gets mad.

T.   What makes him mad then?

J.   We tease him.

T.   Oh you don't? You rotters!

D.   Our big brother b . . . fights us.

J.   Pulled my hair hard today.

T.   What do you do about that? . . . well I spose it's not too bad?

D.+J. (Shake heads.)

T. I'm really sorry to take you out of your Christmas carol practice.

D. I have to, I have to speak next after that.

T. Oh really?

J. Yes.

T. You you have to?

D. Yes.

T. Oh dear! so they'll be waiting for you?

D. Yes.

J. But I think someone else will do it instead.

T. Oh dear! Will that be all right? Do you mind?

D. (Looks doubtful.)

J. No.

T. Sorry about that. What were you going to say?

J. Um. On the hillside outside the town, shepherds were looking after their sheep.

D. That's me. I say that bit.

Family and clinician were satisfied with the outcome of therapy at seven years six months. As the twins neared the top of junior school however they were re-referred for speech therapy due to a habit of pronouncing /s/ with an ingressive air stream. At that time they were criticized rather strongly for their speech at school and were tearful and resentful when seen at the clinic. After further therapy they settled well in comprehensive school. Mother reports that they have no problems with teasing and that they enjoy learning French which she feels is helpful to them.

PETER

Peter, who was under the care of a psychiatrist, entered a special school without speech and with little ability to interact socially at the age of five years. He was not toilet trained and his behaviour was aggressive and unpredictable. Diagnosis was problematic; there were some minor physical disfunctions and the relationship with parents had been difficult and disrupted. I.Q. was difficult to test but was thought to be high. With such a child it was important to concentrate on establishing social interaction and on the pragmatics of communication and language use rather than seeking rapid growth of vocabulary and syntactic skills. It was decided to attempt oral communication before resorting to a sign system.

Treating many years before information on pragmatics became available, the speech therapist advised staff to behave as though the child understood what was said to him and to respond positively to all attempts at communication of whatever kind. It is clear from the transcript that Peter's comprehension level and digital memory span were over-estimated at times but that the avoidance of language drilling and the adoption, at school, of a child-centred approach, together with increased language input and enhanced responding behaviour on the part of all the adults in his environment resulted in the rapid establishment of communication and the use of, and experimentation with, a wide variety of linguistic forms in a variety of situations. Toilet training, which can be seen as an aspect of communicative development, was rapidly achieved and behaviour became socially tolerable, though not exemplary. This child was eventually able to function in mainstream school and transcripts show a steady improvement in linguistic performance, though he is reported to have had greater success with mathematical and scientific subjects than with language based ones. Had therapy been restricted to the use of a language scheme, some of his communicative potential might have been ignored and it is possible that he would have become more dependent on 'taught' structures and more restricted in their use.

Peter now holds a responsible business post, having undertaken a two year technical training for which he required several 'O' level passes (i.e. successful secondary school performance up to age 16).

By the time he had been at special school for six months he had moved from mutism to the level of Transcript 1; his phonology was deviant and his prosody grossly uncontrolled. He was placed, at about this time, in a foster home which undoubtedly contributed to his later communicative development.

Chronological data

By using data our aim here is to illustrate both Peter's improving communication and language skills and the therapist's strategies in conversing with him. As can be seen from the transcripts, Peter moved from minimal, mainly non-verbal, communication to appropriate use of complex grammatical utterances without being exposed to direct language instruction. While Peter does not appear to be pragmatically impaired, it can be seen that his range of pragmatic functions increased over the two-year period of therapy. He seemed to become a more confident conversational participant, as indicated by his questioning and challenging initiations. As for the therapist, she can be seen to use a variety of facilitative strategies such as responding, questioning, commenting, mirroring, correcting, attention directing and explaining.

Peter – March Year I – Age 5;6

Picture-story book I
(+ represents an unintelligible syllable)

P. Oh cold.

T. They won't get cold because it's a summer day in this story. This is a different story about a summer day. Same children.

P. A bottim bot.

T. I don't think their bottoms 'll get cold no.

P. Pant.

T. He's got pants on. She's got a vest on.

P. Botty bot.

T. Yes that's her bottom.

P. +++++ Ruth.

T. Ruth yes.

P. Oh ++ all sand.

T. Yes all sand on the seat what a nuisance.

P. Cold cc oh.

T. He's only got one sock on. He's taken the other one off, and Auntie Jean has bought some ice-cream.

P. Mum +++ (look auntie) Jean.

T. That's Mummy. That's Auntie Jean.

P. A summer summer day.

T. A summer day.

P. ++++.

T. They're all eating their ice-cream and its dripping on the floor isn't it? What a mess.

P. Mummy clean.

T. Mummy's cleaning it.

P. +++. Oh Ruth a got one her.

T. Mm and there's the sand pit for them to play in and all the dolls in their dolls' pram.

P. No more swing.

T. No more swings.

P. Boy running car.

T. That's right he's running to the car. The boy's running to the car.

P. Oh no no.

T. No jumper on. It's too hot for a jumper.

P. A too cold.

T. If the sun's shining it won't be too cold.

P. ++++.

T. They're playing on the floor getting in the way.

P. Get dressed now.

T. That's Grandma.

P. The car.

T. She came in the car. Grandma came in the car.

P. Get get dressed now.

T. That's right she's dressing them isn't she? Ready for lunch. Oh now the men are having some beer to drink. Look, nice cold beer.

T. Whatever's Martin doing?

P. Him. (look at him) (sink)?

T. He's in the sink but what's he doing in the sink?

P. Oh shoes in the ++ (Martin) sink. Mummy++ (say don't) rain.

T. It isn't rain. No it's the hose-pipe.

P. No don't.

T. They want to get cool so they're making themselves all wet with the hose-pipe.

T. Their hair's wet yes.
Ruth's hair's very wet.

T. Well it would be cold if
we did it in the winter
time but it's nice in the
summer time.

T. Now they're having their
lunch. They're having
their dinner.

T. No more swinging no.
They've put the saucepan
on the swing. I don't
know why.

T. It'll go up and down up
and down that's right.

T. I think everybody's going
to sleep now. Oh no
they're going to read the
paper look. All finished.
Now what are you going
to do?

P. H hair.

P. Cold cold.

P. No more swing.

P. Up down updown.

P. Um bottom cold.

P. That one again.

The next transcript begins with a re-telling of the above
picture story.

Peter – September Year II – Age 6;0

P. Get cold why has he
got . . . got pants non?
Why?

T. Well that one's taken his
vest off and that one's
taken the pants off.

T. It was a very hot sunny
Sunday. Let's see what's
happening.

T. No it's midday. No it
isn't its early in the
morning.

T. They're coming in to see

P. Oh why did he take them
off?

P. Let me sit non your lap.
Oo +++ is it night time?

P. They are coming in. Why
are they coming in?

P. Why is the baby maked

what Auntie's got.

T. Well she's joining in
with us. What's auntie
brought for them?

T. Mm.

T. Yes everybody's got
them.

T. They're all dripping all
over the floor.

T. Is it what?

T. Not snow no that's
um they just haven't
bothered to draw the
grass in its supposed
to be a grassy garden.
There's a sandpit.

T. No not yet (T didn't
understand what P was
concerned about).

T. Um.

T. No its stopped you see
Grandma's getting out.

T. She's coming to see the
children.

T. It was so hot.

T. Well he's just forgotten
to put the other one on
or forgotten to take it off,
don't know which. Now
granny's dressing them
properly look.

T. Now uncle's coming with
a duck and a pineapple.

T. Good heavens what's
that naughty boy doing
now?

T. He's sitting in the sink

a little tiny noise?

P. Ice cream. + two ice
cream.

P. + + + + three three. Four.

P. Why?

P. Um is it + there?

P. Snow.

P. Yes + + + has he + (stop)
yet? Not yet.

P. Ah a door a door is open

P. Um why brrrm? (thought
car was moving with
open door)

P. Why is he?

P. Why did he wanted to
take his vest off?

P. Why her has got got one
sock non? Why him has
got?

P. Why are they dressing?

P. Why they are dressed
now?

P. Squirting. Oh why his ee
very naughty?

and squirting water from
the tap.

P. Why his ee squirting it?

T. I don't know. Just for fun
I think. Making a mess
isn't it?

P. Why ++? Why her is
making a noise? (Peter's
attention is being
attracted by a baby in
the room)

T. She's just talking to
herself. She's got to learn
to talk hasn't she? Just
makes little noises to
practise.

P. Don't say that rude word
+? Why did her make
cried last time?

T. She didn't cry very much
did she?

P. Oo a hose pipe. Is it the
hose pipe?

T. mm.

P. Is it?

T. Yes.

P. (One of those that)+++
go round round round
does it?

T. That's right that's the
sort they use for watering
the grass isn't it?
A sprinkler.

P. Why is it a sprinkler?

T. Because they want it to
water a lot of grass and
instead of having a man
standing there doing that
they have one that goes
round and round.

P. Why do they?

T. Because they're clever.

P. Oo why is it the end of a
garden? Why is it end of
a garden?

T. Well we're looking from
the end of the garden to
see what all the people
are doing.

P. Oh why why is the road
there? Why is it there?

T. The road yes that's a
road.

P. +.

T. And that's next door's
garden.

P. A how they walk over
the road do + (round)
in + (down) in there.
Do do they?

T. Yes they do.

T. No I don't think so I don't think the cars go down there do they.

T. It's sort of a path I think. Doesn't look wide enough for cars.

T. What are the children doing now?

T. What are they doing?

T. Just for fun.

T. They might be just holding it up in front of them and talking to each other behind it.

T. Yes in a minute we'll do some of these questions first.

P. Is it a naughty a do that?

P. Yes they do.

P. Um.

P. Reading a newspaper. Why are they reading it?

P. Have. (waits politely)

P. Are we having another book now?

Later

P. Terrible her is a big head. (Discussing the baby) Is it big? Everybody's head's big. Oh her is a messy dribbler.

T. She is a messy dribbler you'll have to wipe her up again.

T. That's it.

T. She's trying to get her teeth to come through you see she bites her finger (laughs) she's starting again now you've wiped her up. You've got all your teeth haven't you?

P. Messy old dribbler. Wipe wipe that.

P. Why ++++ doing?

P. Why her haven't got many? Let me see. Let me see. (laughs)

Peter with foster-mother and foster-sister –
September Year I – Age 6;0

M. What?

                        P. Is Sainsbury's open?

M. Yes. No not on
   a Monday.   P. Why not?

M. Well they have a day off.   P. What doing?

M. Go home and +++ boys   P. No not boys a girls. Not
   and girls.   at mine school.

M. Don't they, well they
   have Mondays,
   Saturdays and Sundays.

S. Budgie come on.   P. Let me feed him.
                          Let me feed him Karen
                          mean.
                          Won't let her me feed
                          him.

S. No I'm not.

M. I think it was Karen's
   turn today. Or is she
   mean?

S. It's my turn.   P. No a her ha h her him
                          should have it in the
                          kitchen really.
                          Should really mummy.
                          (budgie should be fed
                          in the kitchen)

M. Yes I know well we're   P. Why are we treating him
   treating him today.   eat + (mine) his dinner
                          in a dining room?
                          Why are we treat him
                          auntie treat him auntie
                          eat a dinner in here why
                          is why does does why
                          do we?

                        P. Her didn't did an Karen
                          fed me fed him +++ I
                          fed him again.

S. So I feed him tomorrow.   P. No, you won't.

It seems possible that the personal and imaginative functions of language (Halliday 1975) could and should have been taught to this child since there was no evidence of them developing naturally. The interactional and heuristic functions could usefully have moved beyond constant questioning and checking, though it has to be said that simply preventing Peter from asking questions would have been incorrect, if not positively damaging. It is true that excessive use of question forms can obscure some of the problems a child is experiencing. However normal children appear to pass through a stage of incessant questioning and Peter himself outgrew it.

Further examination of the pragmatic ability of this child reveals that having entered school with only a little, non-verbal communication, he rapidly developed the ability to listen and attend, to take turns, to reply, to question, request, respond, initiate, refuse and comment. He used language to enhance his activities, to control others and to defend himself. He mastered the principles of dialogue and his discourse showed some reference to past events and assumed shared knowledge e.g. 'Let's see Jean house'; 'That one again'; 'Is it snow there?'; 'Why did her make cried last time?'; 'Is Sainsbury's open?'

He soon became able to inform himself and others through language and used it to mediate his experience. He became able to participate in educational activities, his vocabulary expanded, his syntactic and phonological abilities progressed rapidly and prosody improved. These appear to have been appropriate goals for language remediation, whereas the ability to reproduce certain prescribed linguistic forms would have been less advantageous. However, there remained some limitations in the child's linguistic skill, which suggests that more attention to linguistic form could have been helpful at some stage and that a *combination of child-centred and language-centred approaches was called for*. There are however so many possible goals for a child with multiple problems that it was thought necessary to avoid imposing limitations upon him by rigidity in teaching.

Although language schemes, for example Derbyshire Language Scheme, (Knowles and Masidlover, 1980) would probably have assisted in expanding this child's knowledge of structures, there remains the question of whether the structures would have been used so adventurously and whether the freedom and enthusiasm with which this child experimented with untaught forms would have been lost if he had not felt himself to be at least partly in control of the interactions with his speech therapist.

There is also the question of whether the fact that 'T' and other staff did not speak to him in 'Motherese' or use shortened forms commensurate with his supposed processing capacity as suggested by Crystal *et al.* (1976) and by Knowles and Masidlover (1980), served to accelerate or retard his progress: on the one hand, he became confused, but on the other hand, he managed to work out a good deal about the rules of language and quickly began to use that knowledge.

In order to judge the level at which this particular child could most helpfully have been addressed, it would have been necessary to find a method of allowing for his apparent grasp of the general drift of lengthy remarks, his successful incorporation of partially understood elements at later dates, his enjoyment of the 'When in doubt guess' strategy (Smith 1983) and the variability of his length of utterance. It would clearly have been unwise to restrict this intelligent child's view of what was possible. It seems likely that some teaching time during which input was restricted to material closer to his own syntactic level would have been useful to him and would not necessarily have inhibited the semantic exploration and experimentation upon which the therapist relied for continued progress. Language drills could well have assisted this particular child's over-all communicative development provided that they had been used in conjunction with other approaches which allowed Peter sufficient opportunity to sustain the interaction himself and to experiment in the presence of an alert and language-aware partner.

Tizard and Hughes (1984) have suggested that because of the confidence usually felt by the child in the home situation and the depth of meaning exchanged at home, mothers have an educational advantage over professionals in regard to language teaching. However, the fact that this child had spent five years in the company of his highly educated mother without developing speech points to the probability that intervention of some kind is essential in some cases. When interraction provides a truly shared and interesting context for language acquisition, the child is enabled to collect language data, initiate topics, ask questions and make comments and demands in much the same way that Tizard and Hughes' sample of children did at home. What is lacking in Peter's case is the use of a 'turn' for more than one utterance except in the case of very casual conversations, for instance the one in the presence of the baby.

Peter – February Year II – Age 6;5

By this stage phonology and prosody had improved very considerably.

T. ++This is a story about these children.
P. Yes.

T. And they live in a place called Paradise Street.
P. Yes. Read it.

T. (reads and shows picture)
P. London doesn't look like that.

T. Doesn't it?
P. No they don't have people like that in London.

T. Don't they?
P. No. (The illustration is partly abstract.)

T. What sort of people do they have in London?
P. Just. Just normalary people.
Just a lot of people.

T. Uh huh well they have children as well though don't they?
P. Yes.

T. And pigeons
P. Yes.

T. ++
P. Are. Are they frightened of London? (Peter is)

T. No they're quite used to all the noise and the traffic they don't mind. Oh there's a horse look.
P. Horse don't look like that.

I've only just seen him
with all those scribbles.

T. Don't they?

P. No.

T. (Reads)

P. Are. Are they frightened
of London? (He is)

T. Can you hear any birds
singing now?

P. Yes. They might fly
in here.

T. What would we do if
they did?

P. Put him out again. When
the window is open + +
bird might fly in.

T. Might it?

P. Yes.

T. Have you had any birds
in the house at home?

P. No.

T. Difficult to catch them
if they get in because
they're so frightened
and flap about a lot.
They hurt themselves
sometimes too.

P. Why do they?

T. Well they fly quickly
around and they bump
into things.

P. What are those two +
(chairs) up there for?
I want to go a toilet.

T. Do you? Come on then.

P. Haven't you finished that
page yet?

T. No we'll leave it open
and then we can see
where to start again.

T. Now then where did
we get to?

P. Do it all over again.

T. I don't think we'll have
time to start all over
again, let's find out
where we were. (Reads
story which concerns
demolition.)

P. Why is it first to
go – number one?

T. Well they had to start
somewhere and they
started at number one.

P. Start + + + + + + (go)

T. Mm they knocked all the
old ones down and built
new ones.

P. Is that a new?

T. Yes.

T. Yes.

P. Is that new?

P. Why did they + + all the old ones down?

T. Well because they were all – shabby and they were falling down and they weren't very nice to live in. So they thought if would be better to build some new flats.

T. But the trouble was you see Charlotte and her mother went to live in a flat at the very very top of a brand new building.

P. Read it.

T. I don't know. We'll find out in a minute. Somewhere up towards the top anyway. (reads)

P. That that one?

T. Well you see her mother couldn't watch her while she played because her mother lived up so high. Is your flat up high or down low?

P. Why do they not play?

T. Oh that's lucky isn't it?

P. Down low.

P. Is, it is a house – actually (maisonette)

T. Is it oh + +?

P. + + + a bungalow on top.

T. Uh huh

P. It is twenty five.

T. Is it.

P. A bottom one is + + seven.
A top one is twenty-nine.

T. I see have you got a garden?

P. Yes it is + (not) nice garden.

T. Is it?

P. No it isn't.

T. Oh it isn't a nice garden oh that's a pity.

P. Is that a moon?

T. No I think it is meant to be the sun.

P. Read it.

T. (Reads, shows picture)

P. They are low. Why does mummy live up live up so high?

T. Well it was bad luck really. She couldn't get one of the flats down low. She had to take one of the higher up ones.

P. How could the children go out a play? (Good question)

T. Well they couldn't you see that was the trouble (reads)

P. Have you read ++++?

T. No not yet. 'Down in Paradise Street Charlie also felt lonely and miserable.'

P. Where is a other one gone to?

T. Other who – what the other child?

P. Yes. Other child.

T. That one yes. She has gone to live up high. That's the one we've just been talking about, she's up high now.

P. Why is she up high now?

T. Because her mother went to live there and she had to go too.

P. Why – why is she, why is he miserable?

T. He's lonely.

P. Why is he miserable?

T. Well because he wants to play with Charlotte and she's not there any more.

P. Where Charlie go?

T. Lets see (reads).

P. Why are they did sing and sing?

T. Because canaries do sing a lot. They just like to.

P. Is that a moon now?

T. Yes I think so do you?

P. Yes.

T. Mm.

P. Have oo tinsd it all that? Have oo finished it?

T. No I've – that was better – I could understand that better when you changed it. (reads)

P. Why ++ hold it by a handle? . . . have you tinsd that page?

T. Yes.

P. Have oo tinsd that? Read it.

T. Sorry, what did you say?

P. Please will you read all that.

T. (reads)

P. Is it time to go?

T. I should think it might
be. It feels like about
time to go yes.   P. No it might not be.
T. Well what shall we do
now then? You can stay
until Gillian comes in if
you like. Do you like
your new class?   P. No.
T. Why not?   P. Cos I don't want to go in
my new class. It doesn't
suit me.
T. It doesn't suit you, why's   P. Read this all about a bird
that then?   one again.
T. That's not the bird one.   P. This was the bird non.
T. It's the snow one.   P. Read me all about no
non.
T. Snow one?   P. Yes.
T. Can you say snow?   P. No.
T. Almost.   P. No book.
T. Listen s – no   P. Snow.
T. Clever boy that's very
good it's called Snowy
Day.   P. Yes.
T. Reads.

SUMMARY

What these clinical examples have in common is an emphasis on communicative use of language and child participation. Lucas (1980) used art-work as a trigger for the
performance of speech acts. In these cases narrative has
been used to encourage the children to make connections
between ideas and to explore events, objects and ideas in
company with a supportive adult (Vygotsky, 1978). The
children are also encouraged to question and comment and
to compare their views with those of others, rather than
to restrict their use of language to predictable utterances.
Narrative is thus employed as a means of building discourse skills and of joining children in their attempt at
making sense of the world (Ellis and Wells, 1980, Smith,

1983, Wells, 1984, Nelson, 1989, Carvie, 1990). The transcripts, even without analysis, serve to illustrate the children's problems and progress. They also provide data for others to explore further.

Chapter 9

Administrative considerations

As we have shown, there is more to communication than correct speech and language and there is more to language use than communication. As human beings we use language in a continuous attempt to explain the world to ourselves and communicate with one another by mobilizing skills and resources of dazzling complexity. Our conviction that speech pathologists should assume responsibility for the facilitation and repair of such a wide range of abilities is based on the fact that, during their training, they acquire more pieces of the puzzle than any other profession. At worst, this breadth of information leads to superficiality or an over-cautious approach, but at best it provides an ability to pin-point and explain problems and to offer relevant assistance to people in communicative difficulties.

CURRENT PRACTICE IN US AND UK

Current practice in speech pathology and therapy reflects society's expectations about correct and acceptable speech and also current developments in the associated disciplines of linguistics, psychology, medicine and education. At times some tension exists between the expectations of a poorly informed public and the aspirations of a developing profession. For instance, therapists may be concerned to foster interactive ability and to conduct research while the initial expectation of clients, families, schools, ward staff and, perhaps most awkwardly, administrators has to do with the correction of pronunciation. Tensions can also result from the conviction of other professionals that their particular viewpoint is the most valuable, the most scientific or the most practical in situations calling for remedial action. Examples of this second type of problem would be criticism from colleagues that currently fashionable or unfashionable concepts or approaches are, or are not, being applied. Why is the therapist teaching, or not teaching, sentence structures? Why is the approach cognitive rather than sociolinguistic?

Unfortunately a feature of the speech pathology field in the 1990s is that it has been under-researched, and as a consequence clinicians are in a weak position when effectiveness measures are needed to justify treatment methods either to themselves or others. For instance, an experienced clinician based in a London hospital recently stated in connection with the evaluation of new equipment: 'It is virtually impossible to access research monies' (Humphreys, 1990, 5). Decisions are frequently based upon the training model to which the clinician was originally exposed and only superficially influenced by more recent thinking. This is because, despite very rapid developments and academic maturation within the profession, updating is haphazard and lacking in supervision and support. Far more serious attempts to tackle this problem can be seen in the US than in the UK. In the UK many therapists do not join the professional association and therefore receive neither a Bulletin nor a Journal. Many lack access to a good library or to adequate courses or cannot reconcile the claims made on their time by a heavy case-load with their own wish to study or engage in research. In these circumstances, how can demands be made that clinicians satisfy minimum requirements for awareness and competence with respect to recent advances? It would be impractical for the same reasons to insist, as is done in the US, that students only receive their clinical training from updated clinicians. Therefore UK students regularly encounter rigid insistence upon approaches and methods which have long been under question from more advanced sections of their profession and can become confused and insecure as a result. Worse still, new approaches can be enthusiastically applied when neither student nor clinician understands the problems or limitations involved.

Some attempt should be made at this point to indicate

the state of the art. If these impressions strike readers as inaccurate, a lively correspondence should ensue which will be reflected in later editions of Clinical Pragmatics. Conversations with academics and perusal of the relevant literature suggest that in the US 'Pragmatics is all the rage'; 'Everybody's into it'; 'One hears nothing else'; 'Pragmatics', is a 'buzz word', a 'band-waggon' etc. When one of the present authors spent time working in California however a different picture was revealed. Not all the clinics visited showed evidence of commitment to communication, inter-action, use of language or contextualized therapy. Other workers, for example teachers and some linguists, regarded speech clinicians as people whose only role was to correct syntax and pronunciation and some influential academics indicated that the introduction of appropriate, interactive therapy was an uphill struggle when working with clinicians whom they did not personally know. In the UK the situation is somewhat different. It has become clear in the course of lecturing to clinicians and students that there is a wide-spread and steadily growing interest in pragmatics and its application to speech therapy. On the other hand, well over 500 clinical supervisory visits have yielded only about a dozen examples of clinicians encouraging students to work in a manner which reflects this interest.

We do not wish to imply that pragmatics-based therapy is good, while treatment which concentrates on linguistic form is not. There may be good reasons for rejecting inter-active approaches in some cases, and there are also under-standable reasons why clinicians have been cautious despite the talk of a revolution (Chapter 2 and Smith, 1988, 1989): speech therapy appears to have been reasonably successful to date. We suggest however that it can be even more so, given the introduction and adoption of properly contex-tualised teaching.

THE NEEDS OF CLIENTS

In structuring services to people with communicative dis-abilities, administrators require insight into the varying needs of client groups. In pragmatic terms, the following type of need can be identified.

1. The confident client who knows that a particular aspect of his or her communicative ability is impaired clearly requires assistance with that particular aspect. The clinician's task is to check the accuracy of the client's perception and to co-operate in the provision of information, strategies, referrals and perhaps a remedial programme.
2. The confident person who is either unaware of any difficulty or only vaguely perceives a problem may become a client because his or her communicative behaviour disturbs other people. In these cases the clinician may be able to adjust the perception of others so that they coincide with that of the 'client'. Either no real problem exists, or it may be determined that there is a difficulty and that it is in everybody's interests to intervene. Intervention in such cases requires care because the client's overriding need is to retain self-esteem while at the same time altering his or her behaviour so as to take account of the needs and attitudes of others.
3. The majority of speech clinicians' clients, however, do not fall into either of the above categories. In the early stages of treatment we observe that a high percentage exhibit low self-esteem, communication phobia, low expectation of success in communication or low interest in language tasks, possibly resulting from the experience of failure. It is debatable whether these clients benefit most from interactive therapy designed to give experiences of communicative success, thus raising motivation and self-esteem, from linguistic exercises designed to improve the likelihood of communicative success in real life interactions, or from some combination of the two approaches. If, as seems likely, it is the combined approach which holds most promise, clients should have available to them skilled clinicians who feel free and able to offer a variety of clinical methods as and when appropriate (Chapter 7). The equipment, premises, policies and attitudes of the remedial agencies should provide clients with the opportunity to receive a combined approach and long overdue research should be facilitated so that what is on offer will no longer be determined solely by preference and promotion within the remedial professions involved.

Furthermore clients have a need, which by this stage in the social evolution of human kind ought to amount to a right, to be treated with courtesy and consideration; to have their point of view respected, though not necessarily agreed with, to receive honest feed-back and information about their communicative attempts and to receive such assistance as may be necessary in making their point of view heard and understood. The pragmatic dimension of treatment is implicated in all these requirements.

In the area of cognition, clients have a need for language as an instrument of thought and understanding and this implies a need for more to be known about the features of linguistic proficiency which contribute to the life of the mind. For instance, is it more valuable to teach children certain concept labels or to encourage them to become skilled at linking ideas and constructing explanations by introducing imaginative play, experimentation and discussion? Should we be content that a person scores highly on a test of comprehension or ought we to be concerned that their comprehension appears to encompass only literal meanings? How valuable is narrative skill to personal thinking or educational success? Questions such as the above are largely concerned with language at the discourse level involving the use of language by the individual for their own purposes, another aspect of pragmatics.

Lastly, we wish to point to clients' need for information, both written and oral, which is presented in a form that communicatively disabled people can process. For example, Government pamphlets and Local Authority literature should be available in a form that does not assume high levels of discourse comprehension; supplementary signing should be available in more situations and should employ a variety of sign systems. It should be more widely appreciated that slowed utterance, visual aids and exaggerated intonation and stress greatly assist comprehension for many individuals. These points refer to the pragmatics of public and educational communication.

It is inappropriate to assume that because the person we are dealing with is a communicatively impaired adult or a young child, no attention need be given to their desires or opinions. Gradually, it is becoming clear in the field of education that tuition arising from the expressed interests and choices of the consumer leads to retention and use of what is taught (Burgess 1986) whereas compelling people to tackle a curriculum derived from what teachers deem to be valuable is useful only to certain types of learner. The same principles apply in the speech clinic (Smith 1988 and 1989). The work of Leonard (1981) (Chapter 7) has confirmed the view that generalization of communication skills will be more likely if patients are not required to be the passive consumers of treatment but are encouraged by responsive therapists to communicate as they learn. Not only will this assist the generalization of skills but a responsible, self-assertive approach to situations and to people will result. Parents of communicatively handicapped children in the UK have recently begun to demand through the Association For All Speech Impaired Children (AFASIC) that their children should not be taught to adopt a passive approach to life but should learn assertiveness skills. Can we assume that assertiveness has to be taught at the last moment when children are ready to become adults? Probably not. Person-centred rather than curriculum-centred approaches to communication disorders such as we have advocated would also be in tune with the thinking of the disability rights movement who stress the need and demand of disabled people to be consulted and informed about their own lives, to be advocates for themselves and to be powerful in the design of their own treatment and the management of their problems (Rose and Black 1985).

THE NEEDS OF PROFESSIONALS

Professionals would like to be clear about their role and the roles of others with whom they work. They would like to work together in personal harmony and to provide an excellent service with predictable outcomes. Unfortunately this is not the picture of present reality in the sphere of communicative disability. In order to move toward the ideal, some of the following needs will have to be met.

Parents will need to be recognized as, in a sense, professional and the status of their profession as one of the most vital in society must be recognized by the community.

Those advising them on the subject of communicative development will need to have a clear understanding of what true language facilitation is and will need to make that knowledge part of education for parenthood as well as part of remedial activity. Care staff at all levels will need to share in this information.

Non-speech specialists such as teachers, doctors, psychiatrists and psychologists will need clear, accessible, succinct and up to date information about what is effective in communication therapy and about the assessments and treatments available. They need, where possible, clear descriptions of problems and explanations of possible causitive and associated factors. Many of the decisions for which they are responsible necessitate this type of awareness and if their sources are not reliable, clients will suffer. These professionals certainly do not need confusing literature about language disordered or language impaired people. There has been too great an eagerness to write about people with communication problems as if they formed a homogeneous group and as a result the literature abounds with statements that can only mislead (Chapter 5, also Leonard 1987). Psychiatrists, psychologists and linguists will need access to speech and language clinics and to language samples and clinical data for research purposes. They also need to know which of their contributions are most valued by speech clinicians and to have opportunities to work in collaboration with them.

All professionals need to maintain job satisfaction. Colleagues need to be able to keep in touch with one another and to communicate effectively. If this is difficult, they need sources of information, advice and reconciliation. Discourse analysis forms part of such a resource by providing frameworks for describing patterns of interaction and methods of conflict-resolution. Speech clinicians/communication therapists need to realize that they have a choice of role and that their training equips them to undertake the latter role not perfectly but at least as well as any other group of workers. As communication specialists they have valuable skills to offer to commerce and industry as well as to people with disabilities. This is crucial since they have a great need for motivating and interesting activity in view of the dissatisfactions currently experienced within the profession on both sides of the Atlantic. They also require the type of updating which clarifies what can be achieved and how. They need clear objectives chosen by themselves in consultation with clients and colleagues. From managers they need permission to do what is necessary for clients and have it funded. If it cannot be funded they need the type of information which will enable them to take steps to improve the situation. Since accountability works in several directions and the provision of a reasonable level of service is expected, evasions such as 'There is no money' cannot be accepted as adequate responses to responsible demands. Clinicians need time, space, equipment, continuing education and support. Above all, they need research time and access to well-researched information which enables them to be realistically accountable. They do not need the type of accountability pressure, too often encountered, which tempts them to teach only what can be easily measured and to substitute a display of pseudo-efficiency for genuine therapy. A further unhelpful pressure is created by the need to show that clients have been discharged, when in fact they require prolonged supervision. This particularly affects children with complex developmental problems.

Administrators responsible for services to the communicatively disabled (if they are not trained speech/language specialists) presumably need clear explanations as to exactly what clinicians are attempting to achieve and what is involved in various treatment approaches. Failing this, they could not be expected to make appropriate provision or to organize lean and efficient services.

SHOWING RESULTS

In order to demonstrate that therapy is effective, it has become customary to rely upon formal assessment materials. In Chapter 6, we have taken a broad view of available pragmatic assessment materials. All of these have their drawbacks where accountability is concerned because of the subjective nature of communicative success. That is to say that if the participants are not becoming more comfortable with interactions, it is inadequate to point to a measured improvement in the pragmatic skills of one of those participants. Only clients and their close associates can tell us whether therapy has brought any real benefit to their lives. Furthermore, premature efforts to establish a baseline from which to judge improvement can distort both the therapeutic relationship and the design of treatment during the crucial early weeks of therapy, at which time many clients experience fundamental changes in self-esteem and communicative confidence. This applies particularly in the case of young poorly communicating children. In the earliest stages of therapy such children can often be observed to respond with a burst of communicative development to reciprocal play with the clinician. Reports from parents that the child appears to have gained confidence and taken a new interest in learning to talk occur too frequently to be ignored. If it is the case that forming a relationship with a skilled and attentive partner can inspire a child to retrace the early stages of communicative development and to experiment with the use of hitherto untried linguistic knowledge, this stage can be seen as fundamental to future development. This would be too valuable to jeopardize in any way. Concentration on language skills combined with a meticulous search for baselines might well interfere with the formation of such a facilitative relationship. For instance, contrast the procedure recommended in Brinton and Fujiki (1989), who provide explicit instructions for establishing baselines in language therapy, with approaches based on personal relationship and interaction. It would be quite incorrect to suggest that gains in specific linguistic skill should not be measured, but it would also be incorrect to attribute only speech and language gains to intervention since changes in confidence or family attitude can constitute the goals of therapy.

It can therefore be suggested that when communicative skills are impaired all assessments, other than those which can be carried out by means of naturalistic observation and questionnaire, be deferred until the client has had the opportunity to benefit from several sessions of high quality personal interaction with the clinician and has begun to behave confidently within that relationship. The benefit will be two-fold. Firstly, it will be possible to gain separate awareness of the benefits of different types of treatment. Secondly, the client will not be misled about the nature of his or her role in the therapy situation or about the type of behaviour expected by the clinician. Early testing and direct instruction can impose a passive role from which it is difficult to release the client when the time is thought right to do so.

When showing results of pragmatically based therapy, one of the most reliable methods of keeping track of alterations in clients' behaviour is video-recording, since this may be subjectively evaluated or used as a basis for various types of analysis.

Finally, it is a mistake to expect treatment always to succeed in conventional terms. Clinicians may struggle to show linguistic improvement in a situation where the client's true need is for acceptance and support. Similarly, persisting with speech or language tuition when what the client needs is play, a communication aid or a personal assistant can be wasteful and unhelpful. Specifying the aims of treatment in broad pragmatic terms in addition to setting more detailed goals provides for realistic accountability.

ACCOUNTABILITY

Given the above, what can reasonably be expected of communication therapists? Clearly the State, institutions and private individuals have a right to expect value for outlay and to reduce time-consuming clinical experimentation to whatever level they find tolerable. However, in negotiating that level, cost-effectiveness has to be balanced against personal and social needs. Resources cannot be withheld to the point where job satisfaction disappears without seriously affecting the quality of service available and clients cannot be denied what they truly require without running the risk of developing further problems, some of which could turn out to be expensive.

Providers of resources ought to expect communciation therapists to improve their clients' confidence in communicating by means of sounds, speech, writing, gesture, sign, or electronic devices. Therapists should be sufficiently experimental to exploit new methods of treatment where possible and they should devise methods of showing how effective treatment has been in moving the client toward communicative competence as jointly defined. Where none of this is possible therapists may well be engaged in activities which assist relatives or care staff to handle, come to terms with or reduce the client's disability or may be engaged in a wide range of preventive activities all of which fall under the heading of clinical pragmatics, in our view, since they help communication to work efficiently.

SUPPORT FOR PRAGMATICALLY BASED THERAPY

Interactive therapy, in which the client is encouraged to take the lead or at least to share it with the clinician, does not appear too impressive to the onlooker. For this reason it is essential to make clear that there is a considerable body of professional opinion which supports this style of treatment. (Lucas, 1980, Craig 1983, Schiefelbusch and Pickar 1984, Simon 1985, Fey 1986, Smith 1988, 1989, Brinton and Fujiki 1989). What appears negligent and unstructured may be exactly what the client most needs at that particular point in order to emancipate him/herself from the passive role and take personal charge of the learning process. Students in training are routinely advised to experiment with this approach and in some institutions are actively encouraged to do so on the grounds that active and highly motivated clients using the therapist as a resource tend to learn rapidly and to use and retain what has been learnt.

SUMMARY AND RECOMMENDATIONS

Current practice in speech pathology tends to be curriculum-centred rather than person-centred but there is considerable interest in the application of insights from the field of pragmatics both clinically and in commercial settings. It is thought that this awareness will improve the generalization of skills which at one time were found to be unused outside the situations in which they were taught (Leonard 1981). This awareness may also improve morale, rewards and job satisfaction among clinicians.

It is necessary and acceptable to clinicians to be account-able to their employers but cost effectiveness is difficult to prove unequivocally when dealing with the most complex of human functions. There are important considerations, other than cost, to be borne in mind such as accountability to the clients themselves.

There is considerable and growing support for pragma-tically based, person-centred, contextualized communication therapy. This is necessarily less structured and more ex-perimental than previous approaches. Such therapy appears likely to meet certain of the needs specified in this chapter. Details of the manner in which this can be brought about appear at earlier stages in the book. Insights from discourse analysis also have their place in meeting the needs described and should be explored as a matter of urgency, for example in the areas of conflict resolution and team-work facilitation.

By explaining pragmatics to colleagues and administrators and specifying their own objectives so that language use is included, speech and language clinicians will make a valu-able contribution to the understanding and alleviation of communicative problems. Teachers, whose approach is fundamentally more geared to pragmatics, will have a valu-able role to play in bringing about change within speech and language remediation.

Managers and administrators need to be fully aware of the implications of changes in emphasis and methods. For example, clinicians may require unfamiliar types of space, equipment and support when changing to pragmatics based therapy.

It will also become essential to review insurance arrange-ments, or to seek family permission for approaches which involve a certain amount of risk, such as conducting therapy or assessment in the supermarket or the playground.

We have attempted to make it clear that if clients are to be enabled to make effective use of new language and com-munication skills, they will have to be allowed and encour-aged to make use of these in interesting and personally relevant situations. To that end, clinicians may wish to share the power they hold during therapy sessions with potentially effective clients, of whatever age and level of ability.

References

Abbeduto, L. and Rosenberg, S. (1987) Linguistic Communication and Mental Retardation, in Rosenberg S. (ed.) *Advances in Applied Psycholinguistics* Vol. 1, Cambridge University Press.

Adams, C. and Bishop D.V.M. (1989) Conversational Characteristics of Children with Semantic-Pragmatic Disorder: Exchange Structure, Turntaking, Repairs and Cohesion, *British Journal of Disorders of Communication*, 24(3), 211–39.

Aune, B. (1970) *Rationalism, Empiricism and Pragmatism: An Introduction*, Random House, New York.

Austin, J.L. (1962) *How to Do Things with Words*, 2nd edn, Oxford University Press.

Baron-Cohen, S., Lesley, A.M. and Frith, U. (1985) Does the autistic child have a theory of mind? *Cognition*, 21, 37–46.

Barthes, R. (1968) *Elements of Semiology* (trans. A. Lavers and C. Smith), Hill and Wang, New York.

Bates, E. (1974) Acquisition of pragmatic competence, *Journal of Child Language*, 1(2), 277–81.

Bates, E. (1976) *Language in Context: The Acquisition of Pragmatics*, Academic Press, New York.

Bates, E., Camaioni, L. and Volterra, V. (1975) The acquisition of performatives prior to speech, *Merril-Palmer Quarterly* 21(3), 205–26.

Bayles, K.A. and Boone, D.R. (1982) The potential of language tasks for identifying senile dementia, *Journal of Speech and Hearing Disorders*, 47(2), 210–17.

Berry, M.F. (1969) *Language Disorders of Children: The Bases and Diagnoses*, Appleton Century Crofts, New York.

Berry, M.F. (1980) *Teaching Linguistically Handicapped Children*, Prentice Hall, New Jersey.

Berry, M.F. and Eisenson, J. (1956) *Speech Disorders: Principles and Practices*, Appleton Century Crofts, New York.

Beveridge, M. and Conti-Ramsden, G. (1987) *Children with Language Disabilities*, Open University Press, Milton Keynes.

Bishop, D.V.M. (1982) Comprehension of spoken, written and signed sentences in childhood language disorders, *Journal of Child Psychology and Psychiatry*, 23(1), 1–20.

Bishop, D.V.M. (1983) *Test for the Reception of Grammar*, NFER-Nelson, Windsor.

Bishop, D.V.M. (1987) The concept of comprehension in language disorder, in *Proceedings of the First International Symposium Specific Speech and Language Disorders in Children*, AFASIC, London.

Bishop, D.V.M. (1989) Autism, Asperger's syndrome and semantic-pragmatic disorder: where are the boundaries? *British Journal of Disorders of Communication*, 24(2), 107–21.

Bishop, D.V.M. and Adams, C. (1989) Conversational characteristics of children with semantic-pragmatic disorders II: What features lead to judgements of inappropriacy? *British Journal of Disorders of Communication*, 24(3), 241–63.

Bishop, D.V.M. and Edmundson, A. (1987) Language impaired 4 year olds: distinguishing transient from persistent impairment, *Journal of Speech and Hearing Disorders*, 52(2), 156–73.

Bishop, D.V.M. and Rosenbloom, L. (1987) Classification of Childhood Language Disorders, in Yule, W. and Rutter, M. (eds) *Language Development and Disorders: Clinics in Developmental Medicine* No. 101–2, Blackwell, Oxford.

Blank, M. and Marquis, A.M. (1987) *Directing Discourse*, Communication Skill Builders, Arizona.

Blom-Cooper, L. (1985) A child in trust, the report of the panel of inquiry into the circumstances surrounding the death of Jasmine Beckford, London Borough of Brent.

Blom-Cooper, L. (1987) A child in mind: protection of children in a responsible society; the report of the commission of inquiry into the circumstances surrounding the death of Kimberly Carlile, London Borough of Greenwich.

Blomert, L., Koster, C., van Mier, H. and Kean, M.L. (1987) Verbal communication abilities of aphasic patients: The everyday language test, *Aphasiology*, 1(6), 463–74.

Bloom, L. and Lahey, M. (1978) Language Development and Language Disorders, Wiley, New York.

Bloomfield, L.(1933) *Language*, Holt, Rinehart, Winston, New York.

Bollingmo, M. and Ottem, E. (1990) Language disorders in pre-schoolers: anamnestic, cognitive and phonological aspects; a paper given at the European Research Group into Child Language Disorders, Norway.

Bonikowska, M.P. (1988) The choice of opting out, *Applied Linguistics*, 9(2), 169–81.

Brinton, B. and Fujiki, M. (1982) A comparison of request-response sequences in the discourse of normal and language-disordered children, *Journal of Speech and Hearing Disorders*, 47, 57–62.

Brinton, B. and Fujiki, M. (1989) *Conversational Management with Language Impaired Children: Pragmatic Assessment and Intervention*, Aspen, Rockville.

Brown, G. (1989) Making sense: The interaction of linguistic expression and contextual information, *Applied Linguistics*, 10(1), 97–108.

Brown, G. and Yule, G. (1983) *Discourse Analysis*, Cambridge University Press.

Brown, P. and Levinson, S. (1978) Universals in language usage; politeness phenomena, in Goody, E. (ed.) *Questions and Politeness: Strategies in Social Interaction*, Cambridge University Press.

Bryan, K.L. (1988) Assessment of language disorders after right hemisphere damage, *British Journal of Disorders of Communication*, 23, 111–25.

Bryan, K.L. (1989) *The Right Hemisphere Language Battery*, Far Communications, Leicester.

Burgess T. (ed.) (1986) *Education for Capability*, NFER-Nelson, Windsor.

Calculator, S.N. and Bedrosian, J.L. (eds) (1988) *Communication Assessment and Intervention for Adults with Mental Retardation*, College-Hill, Boston.

Campbell, T.F. and Shriberg, L.D. (1982) Associations among pragmatic functions, linguistic stress and natural phonological processes in speech delayed children, *Journal of Speech and Hearing Research*, 25, 547–53.

Chapman, R.S. (1978) Comprehension strategies in children, in Kavanaugh, J.F. and Strange, W. (eds) *Speech and Language in the Laboratory, School and Clinic*, MIT Press, Mass.

Chapman, R.S. (1981) Exploring children's communicative intents, in Miller, J.F. (ed.) *Assessing Language Production in Children: Experimental Procedures*, Arnold, London.

Chiat, S. and Hirson, A. (1987) From conceptual intention to utterance: a study of impaired language output in a child with developmental dysphasia, *British Journal of Disorders of Communication*, 22(1), 37–64.

Chomsky, N. (1957) *Syntactic Structures*, Mouton, The Hague.

Chomsky, N. (1965) *Aspects of the Theory of Syntax*, MIT, Mass.

Code, C. (1987) *Language, Aphasia and the Right Hemisphere*, Wiley, Chichester.

Code, C. (1989) Speech automatizations and recurrent utterances, in Code, C. (ed.) *The Characteristics of Aphasia*, Taylor and Francis, London.

Coggins, T. and Carpenter, R. (1981) The communicative intention inventory: A system for coding children's early intentional communication, *Applied Psycholinguistics*, 2, 235–52.

Connolly, J.C. (1984) Speech intelligibility: A clinical linguistic perspective, unpublished paper, Leicester Polytechnic.

Conti-Ramsden, G. and Gunn, M. (1986) The development of conversational disability: A case study, *British Journal of Disorders of Communication*, 21(3), 339–52.

Craig, H.K. (1983) Applications of pragmatic language models for intervention, in Gallagher, T.M. and Prutting, C.A. (eds) *Pragmatic Assessment and Intervention Issues in Language*, College Hill, San Diego.

Craig, R.T. and Tracy, K. (1983) *Conversational Coherence: Form, Structure and Strategy*, Sage Publications, USA.

Corsaro, W.A. (1977) The clarification request as a feature of adult interactive styles with young children, *Language in Society*, 6, 183–207.

Coulthard, M. (1985) *An Introduction to Discourse Analysis*, new edn, Longman, London.

Coulthard, M. and Brazil, D. (1981) Exchange structure, in Coulthard, M. and Montgomery, M. (eds) *Studies in Discourse Analysis*, Routledge, London.

Coupe, J., Barton, L., Barber, M., Collins, L., Levy, D. and Murphy, D. (1985) *Affective Communication Assessment*, Manchester University.

Crystal, D. (1972) The case of linguistics: a prognosis, *British Journal of Disorders of Communication*, 7, 1–16.

Crystal, D. (1981) *Clinical Linguistics*, Arnold, London.

Crystal, D. (1982) *Profiling Linguistic Disability*, Arnold, London.

Crystal, D. (1987) Towards a 'bucket' theory of language disability: taking account of interaction between linguistic levels, *Clinical Linguistics and Phonetics*, 1(1), 7–22.

Crystal, D., Fletcher, P. and Garman, M. (1976) *The Grammatical Analysis of Language Disability*, Arnold, London.

Culloden, M., Hyde-Wright, S. and Shipman, A. (1986) Non-syntactic features of 'semantic-pragmatic' disorders, in *Advances in Working with Language Disordered Children*, I CAN, London.

Curtiss, S. (1977) *Genie: a psycholinguistic study of a modern-day 'wild-child'*, Academic Press, New York.

Curtiss, S. (1981) Dissociations between language and cognition, *Journal of Autism and Developmental Disorders*, 11, 15–30.

Curtiss, S. (1988) Abnormal language acquisition and grammar: Evidence for the modularity of language, in Hyman, L.M. and Li, C.N. (eds) *Language, Speech and Mind*, Routledge, New York.

Damico, J. (1985) Clinical discourse analysis: A functional approach to language assessment, in Simon C. (ed.) *Communication skills and classroom success*, College-Hill, San Diego.

Danes, F. (1974) *Papers in Functional Sentence Perspective*, Mouton, The Hague.

de Beaugrande, R. and Dressler, W. (1981) *Introduction to Text Linguistics*, Longman, London.

Dewart, H. (1989) Investigating comprehension of syntax, Grundy K. (ed.) *Linguistics in Clinical Practice*, Taylor and Francis, London.

Dewart, H. and Summers, S. (1988) *The Pragmatics Profile of Early Communication Skills*, NFER-Nelson, Windsor.

Dijk, T.A. van (1972) *Some Aspects of Text Grammars*, Mouton, The Hague.

Dijk, T.A. van (1985a) *Handbook of Discourse Analysis*: Vol. 1, *Disciplines of Discourse*, Academic Press, London.

Dijk, T.A. van (1985b) *Handbook of Discourse Analysis*: Vol. 2, *Dimensions of Discourse*, Academic Press, London.

Dijk, T.A. van (1985c) *Handbook of Discourse Analysis*: Vol. 3, *Discourse and Dialogue*, Academic Press, London.

Dijk, T.A. van (1985d) *Handbook of Discourse Analysis*: Vol. 4, *Discourse*

Analysis in Society, Academic Press, London.

Dijk, T.A. van (1985e) Introduction: discourse analysis as a new cross-discipline, in van Dijk, T.A. (ed.) *Handbook of Discourse Analysis*, Vol. 1, Academic Press, London.

Dijk, T.A. van (1985f) Introduction: levels and dimensions of discourse analysis, in van Dijk, T.A. (ed.) *Handbook of Discourse Analysis*, Vol. 2, Academic Press, London.

Dik, S. (1978) *Functional Grammar*, Amsterdam, North-Holland.

Donahue, M. (1987) Interaction between linguistic and pragmatic development in learning-disabled children: three views of the state of the union, in Rosenberg, S. (ed.) *Advances in Applied Psycholinguistics* Vol. 1, Cambridge University Press.

Dore, J. (1975) Holophrases, Speech Acts and Language Universals, *Journal of Child Language*, 2(1), 21–40.

Duncan, S. (1972) Some signals and rules for taking turns in Conversation, *Journal of Personality and Social Psychology*, 23(2) 283–92.

Duncan, S. and Fiske, D.W. (1977) *Face-to-Face Interaction: Research Methods and Theory*, Erlbaum, Hillsdale.

Dunn, L.M. (1959) *Peabody Picture Vocabulary Test*, American Guidance Service, Circle Pines.

Eastwood, J. (1988) Qualitative research: An additional research methodology for speech pathology? *British Journal of Disorders of Communication*, 23, 171–84.

Eco, U. (1976) *A Theory of Semiotics*, Indiana University Press, Bloomington.

Edmonson, W. (1981) *Spoken Discourse: A Model for Analysis*, Longman, London.

Elliott, M. (1985a) *Preventing Child Sexual Assault*, Bedford Square Press, London.

Elliott, M. (1985b) *Keeping Safe: A Practical Guide to Talking with Children*, Bedford Square Press, London.

Ellis, R. and Wells, G. (1980) Enabling factors in adult-child discourse, *First Language*, 1(1), 46–62.

Ellis, A.W. and Young, A.W. (1988) *Human Cognitive Neuropsychology*, Lawrence Eribaum Assoc. Publishers, London.

Faerch, C. and Kasper, G. (1983) Plans and strategies in foreign language communication, in Faerch, C. and Kasper, G. (eds) *Strategies in Interlanguage Communication*, Longman, London.

Faerch, C. and Kasper, G. (1984) Pragmatic knowledge: rules and procedures, *Applied Linguistics*, 5(3), 214–25.

Ferrara, A. (1985) Pragmatics, in van Dijk, T.A. (ed.) *Handbook of Discourse Analysis*, Vol. 2, Academic Press, London.

Fey, M.E. (1986) *Language Intervention with Young Children*, College Hill, Boston.

Fey, M.E. and Leonard, L.B. (1983) Pragmatic Skills of Children with Specific Language Impairment, in Gallagher, T. and Prutting, C. (eds) *Pragmatic Assessment and Intervention Issues in Language*, College Hill Press, San Diego.

Fey, M.E., Warr-Leeper, G, Webber, S.A. and Disher, L.M. (1988) Repairing children's repairs: evaluation and facilitation of children's clarification requests and responses, *Topics in Language Disorders*, 8(2), 63–84.

Firth, J.R. (1957) *Papers in Linguistics 1934–51*, Oxford University Press.

Franklin, B. (1986) *The Rights of Children*, Blackwell, Oxford.

Fraser, C.M. and Blockley, J. (1973) *The Language Disordered Child: A New Look at Theory and Treatment*, NFER-Nelson, Windsor.

Friel-Patti, S. and Conti-Ramsden, G. (1984) Discourse development in atypical language learners, in Kuczaj, S.A. (ed.) *Discourse Development: Progress in Cognitive Development Research*, Springer Verlag, New York.

Frith, U. (1989) *Autism: Explaining the Enigma*, Blackwell, Oxford.

Gaag, A. van der (1988) *The Communication Assessment Profile for Adults with Mental Handicap*, Speech Profiles Ltd, London.

Gallagher, T.M. (1983) Pre-assessment: A procedure for accommodating language use variability, in Gallagher, T.M. and Prutting, C.A. (eds) *Pragmatic Assessment and Intervention Issues in Language*, College Hill Press, San Diego.

Gallagher, T.M. and Prutting, C.A. (eds) (1983) *Pragmatic Assessment and Intervention Issues in Language*, College Hill Press, San Diego.

Garvie, E. (1990) *Story as Vehicle*, Multilingual Matters, Clevedon.

Gordon, D. (1990) Propositional coherence in thought-disordered schizophrenic and non-schizophrenic discourse: A listener's perspective, MSc dissertation, City University, London.

Green, G. (1984) Communication in aphasia therapy: some procedures and issues involved, *British Journal of Disorders of Communication*, 9(1), 35–46.

Gribble, D. (1985) *Considering Children: A Parents' Guide to Progressive Education*, Dorling Kindersley, London.

Grice, P. (1975) Logic and conversation, in Cole P. and Morgan, J. (eds) *Syntax and Semantics III: Speech Acts*, Academic Press, New York.

Grice, P. (1978) Further notes on logic and conversation, in Cole, P. (ed.) *Syntax and Semantics 9: Pragmatics*, Academic Press, New York.

Grunwell, P. (1981) *The Nature of Phonological Disability in Children*, Academic Press, London.

Grunwell, P. (1985) *Phonological Assessment of Child Speech (PACS)*, NFER-Nelson, Windsor.

Grunwell, P. (1987) *Clinical Phonology*, Croom-Helm, London.

Gutfreund, M. (1989) *Bristol Language Development Scales*, NFER-Nelson, Windsor.

Halliday, M.A.K. (1967) Notes on transitivity and theme in English, *Journal of Linguistics*, 3, 37–81; 199–244.

Halliday, M.A.K. (1968) Notes on transitivity and theme in English, *Journal of Linguistics*, 4, 179–215.

Halliday, M.A.K. (1973) *Explorations in the Functions of Language*, Arnold, London.

Halliday, M.A.K. (1975) *Learning How to Mean*, Arnold, London.

Halliday, M.A.K. (1985) An Introduction to Functional Grammar,

Arnold, London.

Halliday, M.A.K. and Hasan, R. (1976) *Cohesion in English*, Longman, London.

Hassibi, M. and Breuer, H. Jnr. (1980) Disordered thinking and communication in child, Plenum Press, New York.

Hawkins, P. (1989) Discourse aphasia, in Grunwell, P. and James, A. (eds) *The Functional Evaluation of Language Disorders*, Croom-Helm, London.

Hemmings, R. (1972) *Fifty Years of Freedom: A Study of the Development of the Ideas of A.S. Neill*, Allen and Unwin, London.

Heublein, E.A. and Bate, C.P. (1988) Procedures for a descriptive analysis of intention, *Seminars in Speech and Language*, 9(1), 37–44.

Hoey, M. (1983) On the Surface of Discourse, Allen and Unwin, London.

Holland, A.L. (1980) *Communicative Abilities in Daily Living*, University Park Press, Baltimore.

Holt, J. (1982) *How Children Fail*, Penguin, Harmondsworth.

Holt, J. (1984) *How Children Learn*, Penguin, Harmondsworth.

Howlin, P. (1987) Asperger's syndrome – does it exist and what can be done about it? *Proceedings of the First International Symposium Specific Speech and Language Disorders in Children*, AFASIC, London.

Hughes, D.L. (1985) *Language Treatment and Generalization*, Taylor and Francis, London.

Hughes, S. (1981) *Up and Up*, Armada, London.

Humphreys, C. (1990) The lingual contact sensor, *Bulletin of the College of Speech Therapists*, 459, 5.

Hymes, D. (1971) Sociolinguistics and the ethnography of speaking, in Ardener E. (ed.) *Social Anthropology and Linguistics; Association of Social Anthropologists Monograph No. 10*, Tavistock, London.

Hymes, D. (1972a) On communicative competence, in Pride, J.B. and Holmes, J. (eds) *Sociolinguistics*, Penguin, London.

Hymes, D. (1972b) Models of the Interaction of Language and Social Life, in Gumperz, J. and Hymes, D. (eds) *Directions in Sociolinguistics*, Holt, Rinehart and Winston, New York.

Ingram, D. (1976) *Phonological Disability in Children*, Arnold, London.

Innis, R.E. (1985) *Semiotics: An Introductory Anthology*, Hutchinson, London.

Jefferson, G. (1972) Side sequences, in Sudnow, D. (ed.) *Studies in Social Interaction*, Free Press, New York.

Johnston, E.B. (1980) Communication Abilities Test, unpublished Doctoral thesis, University of Cincinnati, Ohio.

Johnston, E.B., Weinrich, B.D. and Johnson, A.R. (1984) *A Sourcebook of Pragmatic Activities*, Communication Skill Builders, Arizona.

Johnston, J. (1983) What is language intervention? The role of theory, in Miller J., Yoder, D. and Schiefelbusch, R. (eds) *Contemporary Issues in Language Intervention*, American Speech and Hearing Association, Rockville.

Johnston, J.R. (1985) The discourse symptoms of developmental disorders, in Dijk, T.A. van (ed.) *Handbook of Discourse Analysis* Vol. 3, Academic Press, London.

Jones, S., Smedley, M. and Jennings, M. (1986) Case study: A child with a high level language disorder characterized by syntactic, semantic and pragmatic difficulties, in *Advances in Working with Language Disordered Children*, I CAN, London.

Jordan, R. (1989) An experimental comparison of the understanding and use of speaker-addressee personal pronouns in autistic children, *British Journal of Disorders of Communication*, 24(2), 169–80.

Keenan, E.L. (1971) Two kinds of presupposition in natural language, in Fillmore, C.J. and Langendoen, D.T. (eds) *Studies in Linguistic Semantics*, Holt, New York.

Kendon, A. (1967) Some functions of gaze direction in social interaction, *Acta Psychologica*, 26, 22–63.

Kiernan, C. and Reid, B. (1987) *Pre-Verbal Communication Schedule*, NFER-Nelson, Windsor.

King, F. (1989) Assessment of pragmatic skills, *Child Language Teaching and Therapy*, 5(2), 191–201.

Kirchner, D.M. and Prutting, C.A. (1989) Pragmatic criteria for communicative competence, *Seminars in Speech and Language*, 10(1), 42–50.

Knowles, W. and Masidlover, M. (1980) Derbyshire Language Scheme, Derbyshire County Council.

Kress, G. (1982) *Learning to Write*, Routledge and Kegan, London.

Labov, W. and Fanshel, D. (1977) *Therapeutic Discourse: Psychotherapy as Conversation*, Academic Press, New York.

Landells, J. (1989) Assessment of semantics, in Grundy, K. (ed.) *Linguistics in Clinical Practice*, Taylor and Francis, London.

Lee, L. (1969) *The North Western Syntax Screening Test*, North Western University Press, Evanston.

Lee, L. (1974) *Developmental Sentence Analysis*, North Western University Press, Evanston.

Leech, G.N. (1983) *Principles of Pragmatics*, Longman, London.

Leinonen, E. (1990) Functional motivation in phonological development, paper given at the European Research Group in Child Language Disorders, Norway.

Leinonen E. (1991) Functional considerations in phonological assessment of child speech in *Phonological Disorders in Children: Theory, Research and Practice*, (ed. M. Yavas), Routledge, London.

Leinonen, E. and Smith, B.R. (1989) It takes at least two to tango: understanding children's communicative success and failure; paper given at the Child Language Seminar, Hatfield Polytechnic.

Leinonen-Davies, E. (1984) Towards 'textual error analysis' with special reference to Finnish learners of English, unpublished MPhil thesis, University of Exeter.

Leinonen-Davies, E. (1987) Assessing the functional adequacy of children's phonological systems, unpublished PhD thesis, Leicester Polytechnic.

Leinonen-Davies, E. (1988a) Assessing the functional adequacy of children's phonological systems, *Clinical Linguistics and Phonetics*, 2(4), 257–70.

Leinonen-Davies, E. (1988b) Textual deviance in foreign learner compositions, in Turney, A. (ed.) *Applied Text Linguistics*,

University of Exeter Press.

Leith, W.R. (1984) *Handbook of Clinical Methods in Communication Disorders*, NFER-Nelson, Windsor.

Leonard, L.B. (1981) Facilitating linguistic skills in children with specific language impairment, *Applied Psycholinguistics*, 2(2), 89–118.

Leonard, L.B. (1987) Is specific language impairment a useful construct? in Rosenberg, S. (ed.) *Advances in Applied Psycholinguistics* Vol. 1, Cambridge University Press.

Lesser, R. and Milroy, L. (1987) Two frontiers in aphasia therapy, *Bulletin of The College of Speech Therapists*, 420, 1–4.

Letts, C. (1985) Linguistic interaction in the clinic – How do therapists do therapy, *Child Language Teaching and Therapy*, 1(3), 321–31.

Letts, C. (1989) Exploring therapy and classroom interaction, in Grunwell, P. and James, A. (eds) *The Functional Evaluation of Language Disorders*, Croom-Helm, London.

Levinson, S.C. (1983) *Pragmatics*, Cambridge University Press.

Lindley, R. (1986) *Autonomy*, MacMillan, London.

Lomas, J., Pickard, L., Bester, S., Elbard, H., Finlayson, A. and Zoghaib, C. (1989) The communicative effectiveness index: communication measure for adult aphasia, *Journal of Speech and Hearing Disorders*, 54(1), 113–24.

Longacre, R.E. (1979) The Paragraph as a Grammatical Unit, in Givon, T. (ed.) *On Understanding Grammar*, Academic Press, New York.

Lucas, E.V. (1980) *Semantic and Pragmatic Language Disorders: Assessment and Remediation*, Aspen, Rockville.

Lucas Arwood, E.V. (1983) *Pragmatism: Theory and Application*, Aspen, Rockville.

Lund, N.J. and Duchan, J.F. (1983) *Assessing Children's Language in Naturalistic Contexts*, Prentice Hall, New Jersey.

Lyons, J. (1977) *Semantics*; Vols 1 and 2, Cambridge University Press.

MacLaughlin, M.L. (1984) *Conversation: How Talk is Organized*, Sage Publications, USA.

McGregor, G. (ed.) (1986) *Language for Hearers*, Pergamon Press, Oxford.

McTear, M. (1984) Structure and process in children's conversational development, in Kuczaj, S.A. (ed.) *Discourse Development: Progress in Cognitive Development Research*, Springer-Verlag, New York.

McTear, M. (1985a) *Children's Conversations*, Blackwell, Oxford.

McTear, M. (1985b) Pragmatic disorders: a question of direction, *British Journal of Disorders of Communication*, 20(2), 119–27.

McTear, M. (1985c) Pragmatic disorders: a case study of conversational disability, *British Journal of Disorders of Communication*, 20(2), 129–42.

McTear, M. and Conti-Ramsden, G. (1989) Assessment of pragmatics, in K. Grundy (ed.) *Linguistics in Clinical Practice*, Taylor and Francis, London.

Miller, A. (1981) *The Drama of Being a Child*, Basic Books Inc., New York.

Miller, A. (1983) *For Your Own Good: Hidden Cruelty in Child Rearing and the Roots of Violence*, Virago, London.

Miller, G. (1951) *Language and Communication*, McGraw-Hill, New York.

Miller, J.F. (ed.) (1981) *Assessing Language Production in Children: Experimental Procedures*, Arnold, London.

Miller, J.F., Chapman, R.S., Branston, M. and Reichle, J. (1980) Language comprehension in sensory stages 5 and 6, *Journal of Speech and Hearing Research*, 23, 284–311.

Miller, N. (1989) Strategies of language use in assessment and therapy for acquired dysphasia, Grunwell, P. and James, A. (eds) *The Functional Evaluation of Language Disorder*, Croom-Helm, London.

Morley, M. (1957) *The Development and Disorders of Speech in Childhood*, Churchill Livingstone, Edinburgh.

Morris, C.W. (1938) Foundations of the theory of signs, in Neurath, O., Carnap, R. and Morris, C. (eds) *International Encyclopedia of Unified Science*, Chicago University Press.

Muma, J.R. (1983) Speech and language pathology: emerging clinical expertise in language, in Gallagher, T.M. and Prutting, C.A. (eds) *Pragmatic Assessment and Intervention Issues in Language*, College Hill, San Diego.

Nelson, K. (1989) *Narratives from the Crib*, Harvard Unviersity Press, Mass.

New Collins Concise English Dictionary (1982), Collins and Sons, Glasgow.

Olesen-Fulero, L. (1982) Style and stability in mother conversational behaviour, *Journal of Child Language*, 9, 543–64.

Ottem, E. (1990) An analysis of the WPPSP subtests with reference to language disordered children, National Center of Logopedics; Norway, unpublished manuscript.

Panagos, J.M., Bobkoff, K. and Scott, C.M. (1986) Discourse analysis of language intervention, *Child Language Teaching and Therapy*, 2, 211–29.

Panagos, J.M., Bobkoff-Katz, K., Kovarskey, D. and Prelock, P.A. (1988) The non-verbal component of clinical lessons; *Child Language Teaching and Therapy*, 4(3), 278–96.

Paul, R. and Shriberg, L.D. (1982) Associations between phonology and syntax in speech delayed children, *Journal of Speech and Hearing Research*, 25, 536–47.

Peirce, C.S. (1960) *Collected Papers of Charles Sanders Peirce* Vols 1–8; edited by Hartshorne, C. and Weiss, P., Harward University Press, Mass.

Penn, C. (1988) The profiling of syntax and pragmatics in aphasia, *Clinical Linguistics and Phonetics*, 2(3), 179–207.

Perecman, E. (ed.) (1987) *The Frontal Lobes Revisited*, IRBN Press, New York.

Pringle, K.M. (1975) *The Needs of Children*, Hutchinson, London.

Prinz, P. and Weiner, F. (1987) *The Pragmatics Screening Test*, The Psychological Corporation, Ohio.

Prutting, C.A. and Kirchner, D.M. (1983) Applied Pragmatics, in Gallagher, T.M. and Prutting, C.A. (eds) *Pragmatic Assessment and Intervention Issues in Language*, College Hill, San Diego.

Prutting, C.A. and Kirchner, D.M. (1987) A clinical appraisal of the pragmatic aspects of language, *Journal of Speech and Hearing*

References

Disorders, 52(2), 105–19.

Puckering, C. and Rutter, M. (1987) Environmental influences on language development, in Yule, W. and Rutter, M. (eds) *Language Development and Disorders: Clinics in Developmental Medicine No. 101–2*, Blackwell, Oxford.

Pugh, G. and De'Ath, E. (1984) *The Needs of Parents: Practice and Policy in Parent Education*, National Children's Bureau, London.

Quirk, R. (1972) *Speech Therapy Services*, Her Majesty's Stationary Office, London.

Radford, A. (1988) *Transformational Generative Grammar: First Course*, Cambridge University Press.

Rapin, I. and Allen, D. (1983) Developmental language disorders: nosologic considerations, in Kirk, U. (ed.) *Neuropsychology of Language, Reading and Spelling*, Academic Press, New York.

Rapin, I. and Allen, D. (1987) Developmental dysphasia and autism in pre-school children: characteristics and sub-types, in *Proceedings of the First International Symposium on Specific Speech and Language Disorders in Children*, AFASIC, London.

Renfrew, C. (1969) *The Bus Story*, Renfrew, Oxford.

Renfrew, C. and Murphy, K. (1964) *The Child Who Does Not Talk*, Spastic International, London.

Reynell, J. (1977) *Reynell Developmental Language Scales*, NFER-Nelson, Windsor.

Riper, C. van (1939) *Speech Correction: Principles and Methods*, Prentice Hall, New York.

Ripich, D.N. and Panagos, J.M. (1985) Accessing children's knowledge of sociolinguistic rules for speech therapy lessons, *Journal of Speech and Hearing Disorders*, 50, 335–46.

Ripich, D.N. and Spinelli, F.M. (1985) An ethnographic approach to assessment and intervention, in Ripich, D.N. and Spinelli, F.M. (eds) *School Discourse Problems*, Taylor and Francis, London.

Rochester, S. and Martin, J.R. (1979) *Grazy Talk: A Study of the Discourse of Schizophrenic Speakers*, Plenum Press, New York.

Rogers, C. (1969) *Freedom to Learn*, Charles Merrill, Ohio.

Rose, S.M. and Black, B.L. (1985) *Advocacy and Empowerment: Mental Health Care in the Community*, Routledge and Kegan, Boston.

Rosenbeck, J.C., La Pointe, L.L. and Wertz, R. (1989) *Aphasia: A Clinical Approach*, College Hill Press, Boston.

Roth, F. and Spekman, N. (1984a) Assessing the pragmatic abilities of children part 1: Organizational framework and assessment parameters, *Journal of Speech and Hearing Disorders*, 49(1), 2–11.

Roth, F. and Spekman, N. (1984b) Assessing the pragmatic abilities of children part 2: Guidelines, considerations and specific evaluation procedures, *Journal of Speech and Hearing Disorders*, 49(1), 12–17.

Russell, J. and Gibson, M. (1985) When research fails: Implications for speech language pathologists, *Australian Journal of Human Communication Disorders*, 13, 24–29.

Rutter, M. (1978) Diagnosis and definition, in Rutter, M. and Schopler, E. (eds) *Autism: A Reappraisal of Concepts and Treatment*, Plenum Press, New York.

Rutter, M. (1989) Annotation: child psychiatric disorders in ICD-10, *Journal of Child Psychology and Psychiatry*, 30(4), 499–513.

Sacks, H., Schegloff, E. and Jefferson, G. (1974) A simplest systematics for the organization of turn-taking in conversation, *Language*, 50, 696–735.

Sarno, M.T. (1969) *The Functional Communication Profile*, Institute of Rehabilitation Medicine, New York University Medical Centre.

Schegloff, E.A. (1972) Notes on a conversational practice: formulating place, in Sudnow, D. (ed.) *Studies in Social Interaction*, Free Press, New York.

Schiefelbusch, R.L. and Pickar, J. (eds) (1984) *The Acquisition of Communicative Competence*, University Park Press, Baltimore.

Schwartz, S. (1982) Is there a schizophrenic language? *Behavioural and Brain Sciences*, 5, 579–626.

Scott, S., Caird, F.I. and Williams, B.O. (1985) *Communication in Parkinson's Disease*, Croom-Helm, London.

Searle, J. (1969) *Speech Acts*, Cambridge University Press.

Selinker, L. (1972) Interlanguage, *IRAL*, 10(3), 219–31.

Shannon, C. and Weaver, W. (1949) *The Mathematical Theory of Communication*, University of Illinois Press, Urbana.

Shulman, B.B. (1985) *Test of Pragmatic Skills*, Communication Skill Builders, Arizona.

Simon, C.S. (1980) *Communicative Competence: A Functional-Pragmatic Approach to Language Therapy*, Communication Skill Builders, Arizona.

Simon, C. (ed.) (1985) *Communication Skills and Classroom Success: Therapy Methodologies for Language-Learning Disabled Students*, Taylor and Francis, London.

Simon, C.S. (1986) *Evaluating Communicative Competence: A Functional Pragmatic Procedure*, Communication Skill Builders, Arizona.

Sinclair, J.M. and Coulthard, M. (1975) *Towards an Analysis of Discourse: The English Used by Teachers and Pupils*, Oxford University Press.

Skinner, C., Wirz, S., Thompson, I. and Davidson, J. (1984) *Edinburgh Functional Communication Profile*, Winslow Press, Winslow.

Smedley, M. (1989) Semantic-pragmatic language disorder: A description with some practical suggestions for teachers, *Child Language Teaching and Therapy*, 5(2), 174–90.

Smith, B.R. (1983) When in doubt guess: an approach to language facilitation, paper given at British Association for Applied Linguistic Conference, Leicester Polytechnic.

Smith, B.R. (1987) Assessing interaction: The interactive record, paper given at the First International Symposium Specific Speech and Language Disorders in Children, University of Reading.

Smith, B.R. (1988) Pragmatics and Speech Pathology, in Ball, M.J. (ed.) *Theoretical Linguistics and Disordered Language*, Croom-Helm, London.

Smith, B.R. (1989) Communication therapy: The application of pragmatics and discourse analysis to the work of speech pathologists, in Grunwell, P. and James, A. (eds) *The Functional*

Evaluation of Language Disorders, Croom-Helm, London.

Smith, L. (1985) Communicative activities of dysphasic adults; A survey, *British Journal of Disorders of Communication*, 20(1), 31–44.

Snow, C.E. (1979) Conversations with children, in Fletcher, P. and Garman, M. (eds) *Language Acquisition*, Cambridge University Press.

Snow, C.E. (1984) Parent-child interaction and the development of communicative ability, in Schiefelbusch, R.L. and Pickar, J. (eds) *The Acquisition of Communicative Competence*, University Park Press, Baltimore.

Sorensen, V. (1981) Coherence as a pragmatic concept, in Parret, H., Sbisa, M. and Verschueren, J. (eds) *Possibilities and Limitations in Pragmatics*, John Benjamins, Amsterdam.

Spence, L., Fleetwood, A., Geliot, J., Wrench, B., Earles, L. and Searby, C. (1989) A descriptive study of a sub-group of Moor House School children with high level semantic difficulties, in Grunwell, P. and James, A. (eds) *The Functional Evaluation of Language Disorders*, Croom-Helm, London.

Sperber, D. and Wilson, D. (1986) *Relevance: Communication and Cognition*, Blackwell, Oxford.

Steckol, D. (1983) Are we training young language delayed children for future academic failure? in Winitz, H. (ed.) *Treating Language Disorders*, University Park Press, Baltimore.

Stallibrass, A. (1977) *The Self Respecting Child: A Study of Children's Play and Development*, Pelican, Aylesbury.

Stoel-Gammon, C. and Dunn, C. (1985) *Normal and Disordered Phonology in Children*, University Park Press, Baltimore.

Stott, D.A. (1966) *Studies of Troublesome Children*, Tavistock, London.

Strawson, P.F. (1952) *Introduction to Logical Theory*, London, Methuen.

Strike, K. (1982) *Liberty and Learning*, Martin Robertson, Oxford.

Stubbs, M. (1983) *Discourse Analysis: The Sociolinguistic Analysis of Natural Language*, Blackwell, Oxford.

Tarone, E. (1983) Some thoughts on the notion of communication strategy, in Faerch, C. and Kasper, G. (eds) *Strategies in Interlanguage Communication*, Longman, London.

Tarone, E., Cohen, A.D. and Dumas, G. (1976) A close look at some interlanguage terminology: A framework for communication strategies, *Working Papers in Bilingualism*, 9, 76–90.

Taylor, D.S. (1988) The meaning and use of the term competence in linguistics, *Applied Linguistics*, 9(2), 148–68.

Taylor, T.J. and Cameron, D. (1987) *Analysing Conversation: Rules and Units in the Structure of Talk*, Pergamon, Oxford.

Tizard, B. and Hughes, M. (1984) Young Children Learning: Talking and thinking at home and at school, Fontana, London.

Tough, J. (1973) *Focus on Meaning*, Allen and Unwin, London.

Tough, J. (1976) *Listening to Children Talking: A Guide to the Appraisal of Children's Use of Language*, Ward Lock, London.

Tough, J. (1977a) *The Development of Meaning: A Study of Children's Use of language*, Allen and Unwin, London.

Tough, J. (1977b) *Talking and Learning: A Guide to Fostering Communication Skills in Nursery and Infant Schools*, Ward Lock, London.

Ulatowska, H.K. and Bond, S.A. (1983) Aphasia: discourse considerations, *Topics in Language Disorders*, 3(4), 21–48.

Verschueren, J. (1987) Concluding Round Table: 1987 International Pragmatics Conference, *International Pragmatics Association Working Document No. 2*, Belgium.

Vygotsky, L.S. (1978) *Mind in Society*, Harvard University Press, Mass.

Wardhaugh, R. (1985) *How Conversation Works*, Blackwell, Oxford.

Waterson, N. (1978) Growth of complexity in phonological development, in Waterson, N. and Snow, C. (eds) *The Development of Communication*, Wiley, Chichester.

Weintraub, S. and Mesulam, M.M. (1983) Developmental learning disabilities of the right hemisphere: Emotional, interpersonal and cognitive components, *Archives of Neurology*, 40, 463–8.

Weiss, R. (1981) INREAL intervention for language handicapped and bilingual children, *Journal of the Division of Early Childhood*, 4, 40–51.

Wells, G. (1984) *Language Development in the Preschool Years*, Cambridge University Press.

Westby, C.E., van Dongen, R. and Maggart, Z. (1989) Assessing Narrative Competence, *Seminars in Speech and Language*, 10(1), 63–76.

Wetherby, A.M. and Prizant, B.M. (1989) The expression of communicative intent: Assessment quidelines, *Seminars in Speech and Language*, 10(1), 77–91.

Wiig, E. and Semel, E. (1984) *Language Assessment and Intervention* (2nd edn), Merrill, Ohio.

Wing, L. (1988) The continuum of autistic characteristics, in Schopler, E. and Mesibov, G.B. (eds) *Diagnosis and Assessment in Autism*, Plenum, New York.

Wirz, S. (1981) The pragmatics of language and the mentally handicapped, in Fraser, W. and Grieve, R. (eds) *Communicating with Normal and Retarded Children*, John Wright, Bristol.

Wittgenstein, L. (1958) *Philosophical Investigations*, Blackwell, Oxford.

Yule, W. and Rutter, M. (1987) Language Development and Disorders: *Clinics in Developmental Medicine No. 101–2*, Blackwell, Oxford.

Zimmerman, D. and West, C. (1975) Sex roles, interruptions and silences in conversation, in Thorne, B. and Henley, N. (eds) *Language and Sex: Differences and Dominance*, Newbury House, Rowley, Mass.

Subject index

Author index